TALENT DEVELOPMENT IN PARALYMPIC SPORT: RESEARCHER AND PRACTITIONER PERSPECTIVES

Identifying and developing talented athletes to their fullest potential is a central concern of sports scientists, sports coaches, and sports policymakers. However, there is very little practical and theoretical knowledge for those working in Paralympic sport. The book collates the state of the science of current knowledge and practice in talent identification and development in this context by capturing international perspectives of current systems and processes.

Written by a team of leading international experts, *Talent Development in Paralympic Sport: Researcher and Practitioner Perspectives* explores key factors and issues in contemporary sport, including:

- the current state of pathways in Paralympic sports across the globe
- designing optimal developmental environments
- long-term modeling of Paralympic athlete development
- understanding the complexity of talent selection in Paralympic sport

With an emphasis on practical implications for all those working in sport, the book offers an authoritative evaluation of the strengths and weaknesses of contemporary systems for identifying and developing talent in Paralympic sport. This is important reading for any student, researcher, practitioner, or coach with an interest in skill acquisition, youth Para sport, elite Paralympic sport, Paralympic sports coaching, Paralympic sports development, sport psychology, skill development, or sports engineering. In addition, there has been interest from universities to offer courses/modules specific to Paralympic sports.

Nima Dehghansai, Ph.D. is an athlete development specialist with Paralympics Australia. His research focuses on identifying factors that can influence the health of the pathway including athlete attraction, recruitment, development, and expertise. He is currently working alongside key Australian stakeholders on various strategies to optimize environments to maximize athlete development for sustained podium success.

Ross A. Pinder, Ph.D. is an experienced skill acquisition specialist with Paralympics Australia, where he leads a team of sports scientists and applied researchers aiming to develop world-leading learning environments. Ross has supported elite coaches and athletes to achieve success at major international events, including the Rio 2016 and Tokyo 2020 Paralympic Games, notably in Para Archery, Para Athletics, Para Cycling, Para Table Tennis, Wheelchair Tennis, and Wheelchair Rugby. He currently supervises several higher degree research students through national and international collaborations.

Joe Baker, Ph.D. is a Professor and Head of the Lifespan Performance Laboratory in the School of Kinesiology and Health Science, at York University, Canada. His research focuses on talent identification, skill acquisition, and athlete development. He also works with elite teams and organizations around the world to optimize athlete performance and development.

TALENT DEVELOPMENT IN PARALYMPIC SPORT: RESEARCHER AND PRACTITIONER PERSPECTIVES

Edited by Nima Dehghansai,
Ross A. Pinder, and Joe Baker

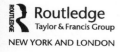

Routledge
Taylor & Francis Group

NEW YORK AND LONDON

Cover image: ©Paralympics Australia. Photo courtesy of
Paralympics Australia

First published 2023
by Routledge
605 Third Avenue, New York, NY 10158

and by Routledge
4 Park Square, Milton Park, Abingdon, Oxon, OX14 4RN

*Routledge is an imprint of the Taylor & Francis Group, an informa
business*

Library of Congress Cataloguing-in-Publication Data
A catalog record for this title has been requested

ISBN: 978-1-032-02647-3 (hbk)
ISBN: 978-1-032-02646-6 (pbk)
ISBN: 978-1-003-18443-0 (ebk)

DOI: 10.4324/9781003184430

Typeset in Times New Roman
by MPS Limited, Dehradun

CONTENTS

FIGURES

TABLES

CONTRIBUTORS

Georgia Askew, Queensland University of Technology and Paralympics Australia, Australia

Joe Baker, PhD, York University, Canada

Eline Blaauw, Gehandicaptensport Nederland, Netherlands

Gary Brickley, PhD, University of Brighton, United Kingdom

Olivia Clare, University of Waikato, New Zealand

Jenny Davey, Canadian Paralympic Committee, Canada

Veerle De Bosscher, PhD, Vrije Universiteit Brussel, Belgium

Sonja de Groot, PhD, Reade, Center for Rehabilitation and Rheumatology, Netherlands, and VU University, Netherlands

Nima Dehghansai, PhD, Paralympics Australia, Australia

Daniel Fortin-Guichard, PhD, Vrije Universiteit Amsterdam, Netherlands

Mike Frogley, Former Canadian Men's National Team Coach, Canada

Adeline Green, Paralympics Australia, Queensland Academy of Sport, and the University of the Sunshine Coast, Australia

Stephen Hadlow, Paralympics Australia, Australia

Gail Hamamoto, BC Wheelchair Sports Association, Canadian Paralympic Committee, World Wheelchair Rugby, Canada

David Haydon, PhD, South Australian Sports Institute, Australia

Colin Higgs, PhD, Memorial University, Canada

David P. Howe, PhD, Western University, Canada

Amy E. Latimer-Cheung, PhD, Queen's University, Canada

Janet Lawson, Queen's University, Canada

David Legg, Mount Royal University, Canada

Hannah MacDougall, PhD, Elite Athlete, AusCycling, Victorian Institute of Sport, Australia

Peta Maloney, PhD, Australian Institute of Sport, Australia

David Mann, Vrije Universiteit Amsterdam, Netherlands

Jeffrey J. Martin, Wayne State University, United States of America

Barry Mason, PhD, Loughborough University, Great Britain Wheelchair Rugby, United Kingdom

Graeme Maw, PhD, Paralympics New Zealand, New Zealand

Alia Mazhar, York University, Canada

Raphael Moreira de Almeida, Brazilian Table Tennis Confederation, Brazil

Krystn Orr, PhD, McMaster University, Special Olympics Ontario, Canada

Raôul R. D. Oudejans, PhD, Vrije Universiteit Amsterdam, Amsterdam Movement Sciences, and Amsterdam University of Applied Sciences, Netherlands

Aurélie Pankowiak, PhD, Victoria University, Australia

Jacqueline M. Patatas, PhD, Vrije Universiteit Brussel, Belgium; BCWSA, Canada

Ross A. Pinder, PhD, Paralympics Australia, Australia

Daniel Powell, British Swimming, Manchester Metropolitan University, United Kingdom

Robert Pritchett, PhD, Central Washington University, United States of America

Eva Prokesova, PhD, Charles University, Czech Republic

Carla Filomena Silva, PhD, Western University, Canada

Jamie Stanley, PhD, South Australian Sports Institute, Australian Cycling Team, University of South Australia, Australia

Ben Stephenson, PhD, Loughborough University, United Kingdom

Robert Townsend, PhD, University of Waikato, New Zealand

Sean Tweedy, PhD, University of Queensland, Australia

Ralf van der Rijst, NOC*NSF, Netherlands

Andy Van Neutegem, PhD, Own the Podium, Canada

Riemer Vegter, PhD, University of Groningen, University Medical Center Groningen the Netherlands, Loughborough University, United Kingdom

Chris Wagg, Boccia UK, British Shooting, English Institute of Sport, United Kingdom

Alexandra J. Walters, Queen's University, Canada

Nick Wattie, PhD, University of Ontario Institute of Technology, Canada

Melissa Wilson, PhD, Swimming Australia, Australia

Michael Woods, Inclusive Sport Design, Australia

Jennifer Wong, Loughborough University, United Kingdom

1

TALENT DEVELOPMENT OPPORTUNITIES AND CHALLENGES IN PARALYMPIC SPORT: AN INTRODUCTION

Ross A. Pinder, Nima Dehghansai, and Joe Baker

Introduction

Identifying and developing talented athletes to their fullest potential is a central concern of coaches, sports scientists, and sports policymakers. However, there is currently limited practical and theoretical knowledge for those working in Paralympic sport. A systematic review by our research team (Dehghansai et al., 2017a), for example, highlighted the clear lack of literature examining athlete development. Subsequent studies (Dehghansai et al., 2017b; Dehghansai & Baker, 2020; Dehghansai et al., 2020, 2022, 2021, Houlihan & Chapman, 2017; Patatas et al., 2020, 2022) from research groups around the world have expanded our understanding, and provided the impetus for this book, which aims to synthesize the most up-to-date research with practice across international Paralympic sport systems (e.g., from those in Australia, Belgium, Brazil, Canada, Czech Republic, United Kingdom, United States, Netherlands, and New Zealand).

As part of Australia's preparation for the Tokyo 2020 Paralympic Games, two of the authors/editors have experienced first-hand the potential opportunities for supporting athlete development. We have witnessed rapid performance trajectories, the quality and passion of coaches and other practitioners working in this field, and the creativity required to solve problems. We also observed (and experienced) many of the challenges that are highlighted and discussed at length throughout this book. We worked closely with sports which, during this period (i.e., 2016–2021), resulted in athletes winning medals at the 2020 Paralympic Games who were not even participating in that sport during the time of the previous Paralympic Games (i.e., Rio 2016 Paralympic Games).

DOI: 10.4324/9781003184430-1

When we reflect on the varied pathways athletes traversed, it is striking how complex these paths to Paralympic success can be as well as the range of opportunities and challenges they provide. We witnessed athletes who had no Para sport experience prior to 2017 qualify for the Games in Tokyo, alongside athletes who were attending their 6th Paralympic Games; athletes who competed for another country prior to the cycle, speaking a different language and coming from a very different culture and system, go on to win medals for their new country; an athlete who was at a recreational level in one sport in 2016, transitioning to a high-performance program in a different sport and winning multiple Paralympic medals. Results were not always positive; there were athletes who retired due to the postponement of the Games who would likely have attended the Games had they gone ahead as planned in 2020. There were also athletes who were 'classed out' (i.e., a shift in the classification system deeming them ineligible to participate) after sacrificing years to their sport. Perhaps, most notably, we saw how this inherent variability and complexity added strain on athletes, coaches, and administrators, a finding which aligns with what we have seen reported in the literature (see Dehghansai et al., 2022; Davis et al., 1993; Fulton et al., 2010; Radtke & Doll-Tepper, 2014).

This book aims to capture current research and practice in talent identification and development in Paralympic sport by harnessing international perspectives of systems and processes. Our own applied work across Australian and Canadian contexts provided the inspiration for this text (i.e., what information do we wish we had to assist us in our work), and our objective was to capture the innovative work happening in elite Paralympic sport, both in the environments we have worked in and others around the world. Some of the questions we had in mind as we considered the development of this text included: What is the state of the talent/athlete development literature in Paralympic sport? What conclusions can be drawn from this literature and/or related non-disabled contexts? What are some of the more unique challenges of Para sport contexts[1]? And, most importantly, how could exploring elite Paralympic contexts better inform and educate coaches, performance specialists, and administrators working in high-performance contexts?

Book outline

The text consists of 13 chapters from world-leading specialists in Para sport. We have attempted to capture a varied international list of contributors from a wide range of academic, applied, and specialist disciplines. With an emphasis on practical implications for those working in sport, the book offers an evaluation of the strengths and weaknesses of contemporary systems for identifying and developing talent. Chapters provide overviews of key research areas and provide calls to action for the Paralympic Movement, practical ideas for sports practitioners, and future research recommendations.

While it was not possible to provide an exhaustive list of disciplines, we have tried to capture the core areas and themes that impact talent identi-fication and development in Paralympic contexts, including considerations for recruitment and identification, challenges associated with classification, the role of the coach, and the potential impact of targeted sports science support. Many of the authors who have contributed chapters here are applied practitioners themselves; however, we have attempted to further strengthen each chapter with a 'practitioner commentary', where we hope to succinctly capture the voice of another applied specialist (e.g., Paralympian, coach, policymaker) from a different Para sport environ-ment, through a short review or reflective piece. We hope this provides readers insight into multiple contexts as well as perspective on how experts in different contexts may observe or evaluate the same ideas and challenges.

After this short introductory chapter, Legg and colleagues (Chapter 2) provide a short historical overview to support our understanding of the background and rationale for the current shift we are seeing in the resourcing and approaches to how we identify, recruit, and develop athletes in Paralympic sport. The next two chapters further explore the concepts of recruitment and development by examining the governance of Para sport organizations (Chapter 3 Patatas & *De Bosscher*) and key considerations on how we can better manage the challenges in recruiting and supporting athletes in the Para context (Chapter 4 by Baker & Mazhar). Wattie and Dehghansai (Chapter 5) then propose new ideas for practitioners responsible for identifying and de-veloping athletes, highlighting the importance of a holistic understanding of athletes' development while taking an individualized approach.

In Chapter 6, Fortin-Guichard and colleagues tackle the critical role of classification and emphasise key concerns of the current system and how these concerns affect athlete recruitment and retention. Indeed, the impact of classification on shaping countries' approaches to recruitment (and the potentially harmful outcomes for some people with impairments exploring sport for the first time) is one of the most critical challenges for the Paralympic Movement as we move forward. Relatedly, Chapter 7 (Walters et al.) provides recommendations for enhancing the quality of participation for all of those exploring Para sport contexts. The authors highlight how practitioners could (and should) strike a balance to reduce the barriers to, and increase the quality of, overall participation.

In Chapter 8, Pinder and colleagues highlight some of the creative ways in which skill acquisition resources have had a big impact on Paralympic programs, and in doing so, provide ideas for how to optimise environments for both coach and athlete development across high-performance domains. Chapter 9 examines talent transfer as one of the key pathways athletes traverse to advance to an elite level in Paralympic sport. Dehghansai and Green present the (albeit limited) literature in this area, highlighting important systemic challenges that persist for athletes and sports involved in transfer initiatives. While we acknowledge there is scant information outside of anecdotal reports or limited non-disabled examples of 'successful' talent transfer, we felt this area requires a lot more focus over the next 5 to 10 years to ensure athletes (and practitioners) are suitably supported to best promote performance and well-being outcomes.

Similarly, another area that requires significant resourcing isPara sport coaching. Chapter 10 focusses on the specific role of the coach in talent identification and development, and (similar to other chapters) laments the over-reliance on literature from non-disabled contexts, which misses many of the nuances and challenges coaches in Paralympic sport may face. Townsend and Clare raise concerns over coach development trajectories akin to the challenges raised regarding athlete development in Chapters 2–4, and subsequently provide collaboration recommendations for researchers and practitioners.

Chapter 11 highlights the role technological advances play in supporting athlete development. de Groot and collaborators demonstrate some of the new (or modifications to existing) technologies used to monitor and track athlete progress and provide robust data (e.g., power, velocity) to influence developmental needs. In Chapter 12, Maloney and colleagues explore physiological aspects of various impairments and how to measure athlete performance considering the variations in many impairments before providing key considerations for practitioners working with athletes that have different types of impairments. Like previous chapters (e.g., Chapter 8 – skill acquisition), a clear message is that harnessing athletes' individuality will contribute to maximizing their potential while decreasing negative developmental consequences.

Martin and Prokesova (Chapter 13) provide some thought-provoking ideas and research in sport psychology, with practical recommendations in areas such as goal setting, mindfulness, and gratitude which could i) enhance performance, and ii) support athlete wellbeing. Some of these recommendations and insights provide opportunities for readers to reflect on challenges raised in earlier chapters. Finally, in Chapter 14, Howe and Silva consider the foundational goals and values of the Paralympic Movement and whether current Paralympic contexts, which emphasize medals and success over participation and wellbeing, reflect these goals and values.

Common themes and next steps

In reviewing and editing these chapters, we identified common themes raised from different perspectives. For example, the need for an approach to athlete development that considered the unique constraints and challenges of the Paralympic and/or Para sport systems was emphasized in several chapters. Similarly, the under-resourced nature of Paralympic sport was identified in several chapters as a key obstacle to athlete development.

Perhaps the most global theme across the text related to the role of classification, which was discussed as a major challenge in the recruitment of athletes (Chapter 4), a key consideration in identifying talent (Chapter 6), central to considerations in talent transfer (Chapter 9) and considered as debilitating to the Paralympic Movement as a whole (Chapter 14). More specifically, within Paralympic contexts, classification was seen as vital to how athletes are identified and recruited as well as to the types of resources provided to athletes, as their classification could dictate how their potential is viewed (e.g., classification depth, their position within the classification system, etc.).

Similarly, elements of classification and impairment are unique to each athlete, thus, approaches to recruitment, support, and transfer (Chapters 3–5, 8–9, 10–13) must account for these factors to optimise development. The unique approach to supporting each athlete is also important to consider when developing athlete development systems in Para sport (Chapter 3), including when we consider recruiting (Chapter 4–6) and transferring athletes (Chapter 9), all the way to how we develop and support athletes through coaching (Chapter 10), skill acquisition (Chapter 8), technology (Chapter 11), physiological (Chapter 12) and psychological support (Chapter 13).

The perspectives of the authors who contributed to this book, and our experiences in field, cement the conclusion that there is no typical, linear pathway to Paralympic athlete development; thus, the critical challenge will continue to be identifying and allocating the appropriate support for athletes who are unique with regards to their sport, their impairment, and their classification, in a broad context of finite resources.

Our aim was to capture the voice of many experts in the field, who work tirelessly to create an environment that is conducive to maximizing athletes' potential. Through these chapters, we hope we have been able to capture the quality and richness of their experiences and the exceptional work they are doing to expand and improve research, practice, and performance in Paralympic sport.

Note

1 For purposes of this book, we utilized International Paralympic Committee's handbook as our guiding working terminology key. As such, impairment was used to describe athletes' biological conditions, while disability was the biopsychosocial interaction that resulted in a constraint for a person with an impairment. Para sport was used to capture the larger Para contexts where individuals with different abilities have the opportunity to participate in sports modified to meet their needs while Paralympic sport focused on the sport settings that align with the Paralympic Games.

References

Davis, R. W., Ferrara, M. S., & Van Nelson, C. (1993). Training profiles of elite wheelchair track athletes. *Journal of Strength and Conditioning Research, 7*(3), 129–132.

Dehghansai, N. & Baker, J. (2020). Searching for Paralympians: Characteristics of participants attending 'search' events. *Adapted Physical Activity Quarterly, 37*(1), 129–138.

Dehghansai, N., Lemez, S., Wattie, N., & Baker, J. (2017a). A systematic review of influences on development of athletes with disabilities. *Adapted Physical Activity Quarterly, 34*(1), 72–90.

Dehghansai, N., Lemez, S., Wattie, N., & Baker, J. (2017b). Training and development of Canadian wheelchair basketball players. *European Journal of Sport Science, 17*(5), 511–518.

Dehghansai, N., Lemez, S., Wattie, N., Pinder, R. A., & Baker, J. (2020). Understanding the development of elite parasport athletes using a constraint-led approach: Considerations for coaches and practitioners. *Frontiers in Psychology, 11*, 2612.

Dehghansai, N., Pinder, R., & Baker, J. (2022). Pathways in Paralympic sport: An in-depth analysis of athletes' developmental trajectories and training histories. *Adapted Physical Activity Quarterly, 39*(1), 37–85.

Dehghansai, N., Pinder, R. & Baker, J. (2021). "Looking for a golden needle in the haystack": Perspectives on talent identification and development in Paralympic sport. *Frontiers in Sports and Active Living: Elite Sports and Performance Enhancement, 3*, 635977.

Fulton, S. K., Pyne, D. B., Hopkins, W. G., & Burkett, B. (2010). Training characteristics of Paralympic swimmers. *Journal of Strength and Conditioning Research, 24*(2), 471–478.

Houlihan, B. & Chapman, P. (2017) Talent identification and development in elite youth disability sport. *Sport in Society, 20*(1), 107–125.

Patatas, J. M., De Bosscher, V., Derom, I., & De Rycke, J. (2020). Managing parasport: An investigation of sport policy factors and stakeholders influencing para-athletes' career pathways. *Sport Management Review, 23*(5), 937–951.

Patatas, J. M., De Bosscher, V., Derom, I., & Winckler, C. (2022). Stakeholders' perceptions of athletic career pathways in Paralympic sport: From participation to excellence. *Sport in Society, 25*(2), 299–320.

Radtke, S., & Doll-Tepper, G. (2014). *A cross-cultural comparison of talent identification and development in Paralympic sports.* Cologne: Sportverlag.

2

PARALYMPIC PATHWAYS

David Legg, Krystn Orr, Jacqueline M. Patatas,
Aurélie Pankowiak, Jennifer Wong, and Colin Higgs
Practitioner Commentary: Gail Hamamoto

Introduction

The performances being witnessed at the Paralympic Games are the result of an evolution in various development systems, of which, for the most part, have not been widely shared (Hutzler et al., 2016). In this chapter, we attempt to address this issue by reviewing Paralympic pathways considerations with mostly using examples from Brazil and Australia, and then reflecting on two pathway systems including those in Canada and Sub-Saharan Africa. Finally, we attempt, where appropriate, to reflect on the remaining gaps and anticipated shifts in current Paralympic athlete pathways.

Development pathways are fluid but for the most part, reflect a system where participants enter, leave, progress, or remain at a particular stage according to their ability, maturation, interest, opportunities, personal circumstances, and/or goals (May, 2020). We will begin this chapter by reviewing recent work by Patatas (2019) and Pankowiak (2020), which brings examples from the Para sport context in Brazil (Patatas, 2019) and from international Paralympic sport expert managers (from the UK, Canada, Australia, and France) respectively. We then present two case studies, one from Canada and the second from Sub-Saharan Africa. Finally, we will argue that due to the multiplicity of Para sport and disability-specific issues, current athlete development pathways derived from non-disabled sport cannot simply be 'copy-pasted'.

Evolution of the Games

Para athlete development pathways evolved after the creation of the Paralympic Games, of which the genesis was following World War II. This

DOI: 10.4324/9781003184430-2

was due to improved evacuation techniques and the invention of Penicillin, which thwarted catastrophic infections, and thus the lifespans of those with spinal cord injuries (SCI) improved dramatically. Thus, rehabilitation took on greater importance and sport was seen to encourage and facilitate a 'return' to society in a more enjoyable and impactful way. Sport competitions were held at Rehabilitation hospitals globally with perhaps the most famous being in Stoke Mandeville, United Kingdom. Here the physiatrist and neuro-surgeon Dr. Ludwig Guttmann hosted an archery competition on the hospital's lawn for 11 war veterans with spinal injuries the same day as the opening ceremony was held for the London 1948 Olympic Games. Guttmann noted that he hoped to one day see this competition evolve into an Olympic-style Games for those with spinal injuries. Twelve years later in Rome in 1960 that dream became a reality.

Originally, the focus of the Paralympic Games was only for those with spinal injuries. Over time, other impairment types were included such as visual impairment, cerebral palsy, and amputations. For example, the first Paralympic Games in 1960 in Rome included only those with SCI but today the Paralympics welcomes ten different impairment types. While the Paralympic Games were at times held in the same country as the Olympic Games, it was not until the 1988 Games in Seoul, Korea that both Games were held in the same city. This practice has remained for both Summer and Winter Paralympic Games and following an agreement signed in 2000 between the International Olympic Committee (IOC) and International Paralympic Committee (IPC), hosting both Games in the same city is now a requirement for bidding.

The evolution of the Paralympic Games has thus been reflected and influenced by athlete pathways. Perhaps this is best understood using three relatively distinct periods as defined by Legg and Steadward (2011). The first is 'burgeoning awareness' which ranges roughly from the Stoke Mandeville Games in the late 1940s to the mid-1980s prior to the Games in Korea. The second era is the 'rise to prominence' ranging from the 1988 Paralympic Games to the early 2000s when the first official contract was signed between the IOC and IPC. The final period is 'transcendence' which reflects the period following the Summer Paralympic Games held in 2000 in Sydney, Australia to the present (Legg & Steadward, 2011).

Burgeoning awareness saw sport for persons with impairments from a purely medical and rehabilitation focus. Here, the purpose of sport was to enable or accelerate the integration of persons with impairments into a non-disabledsociety. Athlete pathways were rehabilitation focused and athletes often competed in multiple sports at any major Games. Rise to prominence then saw the growth of the Paralympic movement organizationally and philosophically. Here was a shift from medical, patient, and disability-based competitions that originated at hospitals, such as Stoke Mandeville, to sport, and athlete-based competitions leading to the creation of the International Paralympic Committee in 1989 (Legg & Steadward, 2011). The pathway systems in some of the contexts during this era evolved with closer ties to the non-disabled sport system where athletes were recruited for and trained for specific sports. Transcendence then saw the integration of athletes with impairments into sport organizations and movements for those who were non-disabled. This occurred at the local, state, national, and international levels including the relationships between the IPC and IOC. In some contexts, the athlete development pathway system also evolved to mimic more closely the non-disabled sport system. This stage is now continuing to evolve with questions related to who can compete in which Games and what constitutes a minimal disability necessitating participation in a disability sport context.

The Paralympic Games has thus come a long way in a relatively short period of time. The Games in its entirety is just over 70 years old and the modern Games, post-1988 is just over 30 years old. The athlete development pathways have also evolved in varying ways depending on the context and we will now review issues facing these pathways systems, noting challenges and opportunities within two different contexts and issues that must be addressed for the future. By recognizing the diversity among the various approaches, we can hopefully better understand the importance of context, the implications for athlete performance, and what pathways may be best for a certain region. In each case, authors with lived experiences will review the pathways noting both strengths and opportunities for change.

Characteristics of Para athlete development pathways

First, we will review a series of issues of athlete pathways. The focus here will be on recent research on Paralympic pathways from grassroots participation to elite sporting success and informed by the views of primary stakeholders including Para athletes, Para coaches, and policymakers (coaches, directors, etc.).

Pankowiak (2020) and Patatas (2019), argue that Para athletes' pathways, should take a multi-level approach to individual development, by highlighting intrapersonal, interpersonal, organizational, and socio-cultural factors influencing Para athlete development. Their analysis is informed by the developmental phases of athlete development as employed in the Patatas et al. (2020, 2022, 2021) studies: attraction, retention, competition, talent identification and development, elite performance, and (voluntary and involuntary) retirement.

There is also growing evidence that athletes with different types and severity of impairments experience significant differences in their developmental trajectories throughout their athletic pathway (Dehghansai et al.,

2017a, 2020a, 2020b; Pankowiak, 2020; Patatas, 2019). More specifically, studies have identified differences in athlete development trajectories between athletes born with an impairment (congenital impairment) and those who acquired an impairment later in life (Dehghansai et al., 2020a, 2020b; Lemez et al., 2020; Patatas et al., 2021). Undeniably, every individual is unique, which will result in different athletic pathways and experiences within these two groups on an individual basis. On that note, these differences are also important to consider when informing programs and policies supporting different stages of Para athlete pathways (e.g., coaching education policies, talent identification and development programs, elite career support policies, etc.) (Arnold et al., 2017; Bundon et al., 2018; Dowling et al., 2018; Kean et al., 2017; Martin, 2015; Pankowiak, 2020; Patatas et al., 2022).

Specific points to consider regarding Para athlete development pathways are highlighted below as a 'snapshot' of how athletes can enter the sport system through sport participation programs and evolve to the elite level:

A. Diverse entry points in sport participation (attraction phase)

For athletes with acquired impairments, the attraction to the sport may occur during the rehabilitation process which is like the pathways found during the Paralympic movement's earliest days. Organizationally, this means that rehabilitation centers and health professionals still have a key role in engaging people with newly acquired impairments. Hence, a collaboration between sporting organizations and rehabilitation programs may enhance the attraction to organized sport (Pankowiak, 2020; Patatas et al., 2022). For people with congenital impairments, the first involvement in sport may be at schools, clubs, or associations that offer Para sport program opportunities (Jeanes et al., 2019; Pankowiak, 2020; Patatas et al., 2022). For example, in Brazil, the most likely place of entry in sport participation for Paralympic athletes is in sport clubs (67%), followed by rehabilitation centers in the case of athletes with an acquired impairment (36%), and specialized clubs for athletes with a congenital impairment (22%). The higher proportion of athletes being attracted to Para sport in sports clubs or rehabilitation centers reinforces the need to develop practical training and qualification for coaches and health personnel involved in the rehabilitation processes (Patatas, 2019).

B. Great age variations of athletes with impairments

Athletes with acquired impairments usually start playing sport at an older age while athletes with congenital impairments start earlier (Patatas et al., 2021).

Indeed, both groups usually start on the pathway at an older starting age than non-disabled athletes, which may be related to the lack of Para sport opportunities in clubs or schools, and/or to negative socio-cultural norms and preconceptions about the involvement of people with disabilities in sport (Pankowiak, 2020; Patatas et al., 2022). In recent studies on Paralympic sport policies, sport managers reported that programming aiming to raise awareness about sport opportunities for people with impairments was critical (Jeanes et al., 2019; Pensgaard & Sorensen, 2002). In terms of sport governance, this also means that it is essential that programs are available and accessible to both children with impairment at school and to adults who are entering Para sport participation later in life, and that coaches are trained in both stages and within the Para sport domain (Pankowiak, 2020; Patatas et al., 2020; Wareham et al., 2018).

C. Duration of the developmental phases

Relative to the pathway of Olympic athletes, the developmental trajectories (from the attraction to the sport to the elite phase) of athletes with impairments are generally shorter (Pankowiak, 2020; Patatas et al., 2022; 2021). This is potentially related, among other reasons, to the relatively small number of competitors per Para sport class (Pankowiak, 2020). In addition, a recent study from Patatas et al. (2021) showed that the pathway to the elite phase of athletes with an acquired impairment is generally shorter (i.e., fast-track) than that of athletes born with an impairment. Athletes that acquired an impairment later in life take approximately 4.5 years to reach the elite phase compared to almost 6 years for athletes with a congenital impairment (Patatas et al., 2021). According to Para sport stakeholders from Brazil, this difference in the duration of an athletic career pathway could be related to several elements. For example, athletes with acquired impairments may develop sporting skills through sport participation before acquiring their impairment and thus are able to transfer those skills to their current Para sport. This hypothesis is supported by the studies of Dehghansai et al. (2017b) and Lemez et al. (2020) suggesting a similar outcome when investigating athletes from Canada.

D. The interconnection between classification, talent identification, and elite development pathways

As talented as an athlete with an impairment may be in a particular sport, if the athlete does not meet the minimum eligibility criteria of the classification system in that sport, this athlete will not be able to enter Paralympic sport classification system unless they have an eligible impairment to be confirmed in a class. This has critical implications for athletes with impairments with the ambition to devote their time and energy to focus on high-performance career development. Classification is a cornerstone of Paralympic sports, as it determines which Para athletes are eligible to compete and in which sport-specific class. As a result, classification is often the entry point into a Paralympic pathway. From an organizational perspective, it is critical for national sporting systems and organizations to develop and implement classification procedures to determine who is eligible to enter a Para sport class as early as possible, to prevent athletes the trauma that can result from being de-classified (Bundon et al., 2018; Dehghansai et al., 2021; Pankowiak, 2020; Patatas et al., 2020).

E. Intermediate phase leading towards talent identification

As the competitive pathway for Para athletes tends to be rapid, their participation in competitions starts relatively early (e.g., at a young age, or relatively rapidly after having acquired an impairment). Para athletes can be identified by national coaches while participating in regional or provincial competitions, or during events specifically organized to detect talented athletes, such as the 'Paralympian search' (Dehghansai & Baker, 2020). During this stage, classifiers are essential stakeholders, specifically ensuring that the national classification process is reliable (i.e., reducing the chances of misclassification) as well as in informing talent identification processes. Due to its nature, the classification system heavily influences the selection of the most competitive talented athletes (Howe & Jones, 2006). As each Para sport class represents a spectrum of impairment severity, within a specific class, an athlete who has one of the most severe degrees of impairment will be less likely to be competitive in that class (Pankowiak, 2020; Patatas et al., 2022). Strategically, in terms of elite sport policies this has several implications, such as the commitment of resources to optimize the development of athletes with less severe impairments in a sport class (Pankowiak, 2020).

F. Athletic career termination and retirement

Some Para athletes are 'forced' to terminate their athletic career due to Para sport-specific reasons, causing an involuntary retirement. Reasons include the impairment progression or changes in classification. Examples of this could be when the athletes' classification or medical condition changes, and the athlete is no longer eligible to compete, or the classification or event is eliminated from the Paralympic program (Bundon et al., 2018; Pankowiak, 2020). To minimize potential trauma that an involuntary or voluntary retirement from an athletic career can cause, and to ensure successful career transitions out of the sport, rigorous classification guidelines and policies aiming to support athlete wellbeing and post-career support are critical (Patatas et al., 2020).

Case studies

The second section of this chapter now provides two case studies of Para athlete development pathways. The first is from Sub-Saharan Africa, which is practical in nature while the second is from Canada and is more theoretical in approach.

Sub-Saharan Africa

Focusing on Sub-Saharan Africa, the first athletes who competed internationally were from South Africa at the Tokyo 1964 Paralympic Games, and later in Kenya 1976 Paralympic Games. However, it was not until 1992 that other countries, including Côte d'Ivoire, Ghana, Sierra Leone, and Zimbabwe made their debut. By the Atlanta 1996 Paralympic Games, over 100 nations from around the world were represented, including six new Sub-Saharan African countries including Angola, Burkina Faso, Nigeria, Mauritius, Uganda, and Zambia. In the 10 years between the Atlanta 1996 Paralympic Games and Rio 2016 Paralympic Games, this number grew to 37 Sub-Saharan African countries, with leading performances and the largest delegations coming from South Africa, Nigeria, and Kenya. Despite this rapid growth in representation, the region has had very little podium success, with 25 countries yet to win a medal.

Many factors have likely influenced why medal performances have not followed the growth in participation and one may be a poorly developed athlete pathway system. This, in turn, has been impacted by many other factors with one of the most prominent perhaps being the stigma associated with disability. The convergence of traditional, cultural, and religious beliefs and influences of colonial and missionary practices of charity and medical segregation, have contributed to stigma that prevents people with impairments from enjoying human rights such as education, health care, employment as well as sport, recreation, and cultural activities (Berghs, 2017; Rohwerder, 2018; Stone-MacDonald, & Butera, 2014). Global instruments such as the World Health Organization International Classification of Functioning, Disability and Health (WHO ICF) and the United Nations Convention on the Rights of Persons with Disabilities (UN CRPD), which advocates for a human-rights centered approach, are slowly influencing public policy and changing perceptions.

Other changes result from the examples of athletes and organizations. In South Africa, for example, long-standing participation and visibility of Paralympians like Natalie DuToit (Seggie, 2012), coupled with the formation of the South African Confederation and Olympic Committee (SASCOC) in 2005, played critical roles in the inclusion of Paralympic athletes within the South African Sport system, especially at the high-performance level. SASCOC is recognized as South Africa's National Paralympic Committee (NPC) and is responsible for delivery of Team South Africa to all multi-sport coded events (i.e., Olympics, Paralympics, Commonwealth Games, etc.). It also takes responsibility for all high-performance sport functions. The South African Sport Association for Physically Disabled (SASAPD), meanwhile, acts as the multisport federation for 9 sports across 9 provinces and has the responsibility for managing the provision of an internationally accredited classification system, competition structures as well as education, training, sport science through collaboration with universities and mass participation (South African Sport Association for the Physically Disabled, 2021). The formation of SASCOC thus helped to clarify responsibilities and recognition of Paralympic sport and its athletes across the national sport structures and the resultant increased visibility continues to aid advocacy efforts for further disability inclusion across all levels of the athlete pathways.

In Kenya and Nigeria, meanwhile, NPCs are responsible for the delivery of their national teams to the Paralympic Games, while the National Olympic Committees assume responsibility for Olympic and Commonwealth Games participation. This is like many other countries and regions with Para sport development thus being the responsibility of NPC sub-committees and member federations. Both Kenya and Nigeria have been successful on the world stage, but unlike South Africa (who have medal success across nine sports), they have focused resources into single sports such as Para Athletics and Para Powerlifting.

The structures seen in Kenya and Nigeria are the most common across the sub-Saharan region. In many developed nations, meanwhile, entry into Para sport is typically through inclusive physical education and school sport for young people or through rehabilitation centers for those acquiring impairments later in life. In Sub-Saharan Africa, however, disability stigma, poverty, and accessibility limit the attendance of young people with impairments to school and access to health care. Consequently, most potential Para athletes are invited into the pathway directly by coaches or through word of mouth. Regular Para sport training is also mostly only available in urban centers but is still limited by equipment, sport-specific assistive technology, facility accessibility and trained coaches.

Other barriers within the pathway process in the Sub-Saharan context and which were highlighted earlier in this chapter are challenges to fulfilling athletes' requirements with international classification. The first step in the classification process is to submit medical documents to the respective international federations and these are usually costly and difficult to navigate within local health systems. The second step is for the athlete to attend a sanctioned competition with international classification. These are sparse in Sub-Saharan Africa, and typically, African championships are held in South Africa or northern African countries due to sport infrastructure. A regular Pan-African Games, meanwhile, does not exist, and as a result, most Sub-Saharan African countries are forced to travel outside of the continent for classification and qualification that is costly and complicated by entry visa requirements.

In summary, many hurdles limit Para sport pathway development in Sub-Saharan Africa. Elevating performances of Para athletes and creating sustainable pathways will thus require further coordination, leadership, and investment across national, continental, and international sport structures. At the high-performance level, policymaking should take a mainstream to disability inclusion approach that would work towards equivalent structures and supports for athletes with and without impairments. Raising the visibility of Para sport and Para athletes across the region through communication channels such as television, radio, social media, and local practices could also play a critical role to reduce stigma, raise visibility and promote investment.

Canada

In this section, we will review the Canadian Long Term Athlete Development model (LTAD). This case study will be more theoretically focused compared to the Sub-Sahara African one that focused more on the practical implications of athlete pathways.

Canada has been developing their Long-Term Development model for athletes, including athletes with an impairment since 2004. This framework was based on work from the 1990s spearheaded by Istvan Baly and Richard Way working originally with Alpine Canada (Skiing).

The Canadian framework produced by the Sport for Life Society, a Canadian non-government organization, has gone through three major editions since its inception. The original, Canadian Sport for life: Long Term Athlete Development did not explicitly include athletes with an impairment and a supplement, No-Accidental Champions, was released in 2006 which focused on athletes with physical and sensory disabilities. Both documents were updated a decade ago and No Accidental Champions was expanded to include athletes with intellectual disabilities.

A major update of Sport for Life's flagship document in 2019, was both a change in name and focus. The latest edition is now called Long-Term Development in Sport and Physical Activity with the name change signaling that long-term development is important not just for high-performance athletes but also for those wanting to engage in life-long physical activity. It also signals that optimum long-term development of

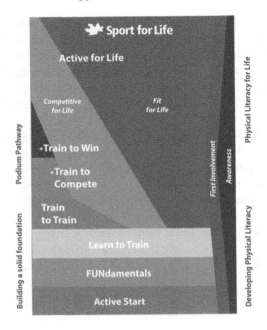

FIGURE 2.1 The Sport for Life Framework for long-term development in sport and physical activity

athletes requires similar long-term development of coaches, officials, and other participants in the sport system.

The Canadian framework (see Figure 2.1), is based on the key idea of exposing children and youth to developmentally appropriate activities at each stage of their development, while building a solid foundation during the first three stages (Active Start: Boys and Girls ages birth to 6. FUNdamentals, Girls 6–8, boys 6–9 and Learn to Train: Girls 8 to onset of adolescent growth spurt, boys 9 to onset). The focus in these stages is on building physical literacy and positive attitudes towards physical activity. The model, as noted earlier, is based on non-disabled contexts but was adapted to incorporate a few disability-specific elements. This model is also potentially applicable for both those with acquired and congenital impairments.

In an ideal context Active Start and FUNdamentals would focus on non-sport-specific development of basic human movements and fundamental movement skills, while Learn to Train would encourage development of a wide range of foundational sport-specific skills such as catching and throwing (i.e., sending and receiving). Throughout these first three stages, participants would be encouraged to engage in active play on the ground, in water, on snow and ice, and in the air.

During Train to Train, the period of adolescent growth, athletes (both non-disabled and those with impairments) are encouraged to develop sport-specific skills. Those with the talent and drive enter their sport's Podium Pathway from the grassroots to high-performance in the Train to Compete and Train to Win stages. Train to Compete athletes are generally at the junior national team level, or equivalent, while Train to Train athletes are competitive at the very highest professional or Olympic/Paralympic level. At any time after Learn to Train, individuals may move to Active for Life where they may continue to compete without aspirations to World Championship level (but may compete at very high master's level) or may take part in their sport for health and/or social reasons. In addition, this pathway also recognizes that to take part in a sport one must be aware of its existence, and that an individual's very first involvement with a sport can have a highly negative or positive impact on their involvement.

As mentioned earlier, this Canadian model was designed to be applied to non-disabled athletes and those with acquired and congenital impairments. For those with an acquired impairment they would be encouraged to follow the same developmentally appropriate framework prior to acquisition and following the acquisition of the impairment they would be encouraged to pass through modified stages of becoming active again, learning fundamental movement skills to the greatest extent possible, learning a range of sport-specific skills before specializing, and then refining their skills and capabilities within the sport of their choice.

Also, and as noted earlier, the theory and practice of this model are sometimes not aligned. Low numbers of athletes with a disability and unevenly distributed opportunities for Para sport across Canada with a massive geographical size means that the development of high-performance athletes with a disability is non-linear and reaching the top in a sport often follows an individual pathway. Regardless, the Canadian pathway can hopefully provide guidance in other contexts recognizing that it will need to be adaptable and flexible to a variety of issues.

After reviewing examples of Para sport athlete development pathways with several global examples and then specific case studies focusing on Canada, and sub-Saharan Africa, the final section of this chapter will address gaps and anticipated shifts. These are both applicable to the nations addressed earlier in this chapter but also likely globally.

Future research

While many gaps exist in the Paralympic athlete pathways, we will focus in this final section on two; mental health and its' impact on the pathway process for athletes with an impairment and improving and expanding the recreational Para sport pathways. Both are underserved in the academic literature and sporting communities and warrant further attention.

Recreational pathways

One area for further consideration is at the recreational level of sport participation. There is a global need for more recreational-level opportunities, and for those programs to be coached by those with Para sport training and more specifically and ideally coaches with an impairment. Recreational opportunities are essential as not everyone is interested in being a Paralympian, but most, if not all, can benefit from the physical and social participation outcomes that Para sports can offer (Orr et al., 2019). For some individuals, sport may be the physical activity they are most motivated by. However, the opportunity to participate in programs that provide quality experiences (Evans et al., 2018) in a need-satisfying and safe environment is not always available.

Furthermore, from the high-performance sport literature, coaches with specialized training and experience as a high-performance athlete have the potential to provide high-quality sport and developmental training to young athletes on the talent pathway (Williams, 2021). However, depending on the country or sport organization, coaches may be volunteers with little or no training, and have various personal experiences in Para sport (Douglas et al., 2018). Having coaches, volunteers, and training staff who have an impairment is especially important during initial involvement with sport as individuals with similar lived experiences can challenge stereotypes and dis/ablism of individuals who identify with an impairment (Richardson et al., 2017).

Mental health

Mental health is a second area that has been underserved in both research and practice for athletes with an impairment (Arnold et al., 2017; Patatas et al., 2020). While non-disabled athletes have engaged in research to understand the stressors of high-performance athletes (Arnold & Fletcher, 2012), less is known about the range and similarity of stressors that athletes with impairments (Arnold et al., 2017). From Arnold and colleagues' (2017) study, 316 sources of stress across 35 categories were identified. For example, the classification process may be beneficial for Para sports on a communal level (Patatas et al., 2020); however, individually, classification can present as a stress-triggering event for athletes and their support network. The classification process is thus a unique stressor to athletes who identify with an impairment. Specifically, classification may be perceived to be unfair, incorrect, changed, or occurring too late in the competition cycle, and not well explained to newer athletes (Arnold et al., 2017). Thus, more work is warranted to explore how to effectively address the complexity of stressors faced by athletes with an impairment.

In addition to the multitude of stressors identified by athletes with impairments, the mental health diagnoses of these athletes are under-represented in the literature. For example, from a Canadian perspective, recent literature suggests that there is no difference in rates of depression, general anxiety disorder, or eating disorders between Canadian Paralympians and Olympians (Poucher et al., 2021), and almost 42% of elite athletes report at least one form of mental health concern (Poucher et al., 2020). The reality, however, is that little literature exists that specifically addresses proactive strategies for promoting mental well-being among athletes with an impairment.

Conclusion

Several frameworks have been developed over the last 20 years to understand athletes' development pathways from sport participation to the elite level (Balyi et al., 2013; Gulbin et al., 2013; Patatas et al., 2022). The few that do exist have been used to inform sport scientists, practitioners, and policymakers working to optimize the development of participants into life-long physically active people and/or elite athletes. In this chapter, we focused on characteristics of the existing development pathways for athletes with impairments from the point where they enter the sport to high-performance Paralympic sport competitions (e.g., IPC Athletics world championship, the Paralympics). To do this we used several national and regional contexts and the chapter concluded with a review of two areas for future research and examination.

The Paralympic Games began officially in 1960 and have evolved to become the second-largest multisport event in the world, along with being the pinnacle of sporting achievement for athletes with impairments. The transformation has seen an evolution from a medical model where sport was used for the purposes of rehabilitation to one focusing on elite athlete performance. Alongside this has been an evolution in athlete pathways (Legg & Steadward, 2011).

Undeniably, every individual is unique, which will result in different athletic pathways and experiences but within these various experiences are common themes which we have tried to identify. Our hope is that by reviewing the creation of a few pathways and recommendations for future research that the development of future pathways will be more effective and efficient.

Practitioner commentary

Ultimately, the success of any pathway in Para sport is dependent on a holistic and participant-centered approach that is capable of providing individualized support in addressing the barriers to participation and progression in the system. In both the Canadian and Sub-Saharan contexts, the diversity and intersectionality of participants with impairments are vast and directly affect their experience of, and access to, sport. Furthermore, the geographic differences within both contexts challenge the effectiveness of a singular pathway for a country as large as Canada, or a continent such as Africa. Pathway models provide the theoretical context and understanding for sport administrators and coaches to ensure the necessary stages and elements exist, however it is humanizing the system that will contribute most to its success.

Therefore, it is critically important for coaches, sport administrators, and organizational leadership to embrace and provide sufficient resources in support of individuals as they navigate the system. This may take the form of peer support from someone with lived experience who not only serves as a role model but can also provide real-life solutions. It may be an equipment loan program at low or no cost to individuals or communities to support the early stages of participation in the pathway. It may be targeting competitions out of the country for classification opportunities and providing the resources to attend, including financial, support personnel, and logistics. It may be acknowledging the mental health supports required and the impact of traumatic injury on their journey through the pathway. It is, most importantly, listening to the voices of the athletes we serve.

All of this requires greater resources and enhanced knowledge as compared to the non-disabled sport system, and as a result, provisions that are 'the same as' or 'equal to' those for nondisabled athletes are insufficient. For an athletic career pathway to result in lifelong participation in Para sport or high-performance athlete success, it must provide equitable opportunities that acknowledge diversity and intersectionality, and not be a passive structure that relies on the participant's ability to navigate the system on their own.

A critical debate affecting pathway models and system alignment is the range of approaches from an integration perspective. Programs, events, and organizations exist on a continuum from disability-specific to fully integrated with non-disabled athletes. Pathways may diverge and converge with a non-disabled system depending on the age and stage of the participant and available opportunities, expertise, and resources in the community. Success of the athlete experience on this continuum is once again centered on how well the pathway and structure are meeting the needs of the participant and most importantly, whether it is adequately resourced and supported, both financially and with knowledgeable, experienced peers, coaches, and administrators.

Advocacy, increased awareness, and greater visibility of Para sport has the power to affect societal change and improve the quality of life of individuals with impairments far beyond sport. As a result, the work of developing pathways takes on even greater importance and weight, and must be both responsive to an ever-evolving sport and social environment and innovative in creating the future we know is possible.

References

Arnold, R. & Fletcher, D. (2012). A research synthesis and taxonomic classification of the organizational stressors encountered by sport performers. *Journal of Sport and Exercise Psychology, 34*, 397–429.

Arnold, R., Wagstaff, C. R. D., Steadman, L., & Pratt, Y. (2017). The organisational stressors encountered by athletes with a disability. *Journal of Sports Sciences, 35*(12), 1187–1196.

Balyi, I., Way, R., & Higgs, C. (2013). *Long-term athlete development.* New York, NY: Human Kinetics.

Berghs, M. (2017). Practices and discourses of ubuntu: Implications for an African model of disability? *African Journal of Disability (Online), 6*(292), 1–8.

Bundon, A., Ashfield, A., Smith, B., & Goosey-Tolfrey, V. L. (2018). Struggling to stay and struggling to leave: The experiences of elite para-athletes at the end of their sport careers. *Psychology of Sport and Exercise, 37*, 296–305.

Dehghansai, N. & Baker, J. (2020). Searching for Paralympians: Characteristics of participants attending "search" events. *Adapted Physical Activity Quarterly, 37*(1), 1–10.

Dehghansai, N., Lemez, S., Wattie, N., & Baker, J. (2017a). Training and development of Canadian wheelchair basketball players. *European Journal of Sport Science, 17*(5), 511–518.

Dehghansai, N., Lemez, S., Wattie, N., & Baker, J. (2017b). A systematic review of influences on development of athletes with disabilities. *Adapted Physical Activity Quarterly, 34*(1), 72–90.

Dehghansai, N., Lemez, S., Wattie, N., Pinder, R. A., & Baker, J. (2020a). Understanding the development of elite parasport athletes using a constraint-led approach: Considerations for coaches and practitioners. *Frontiers in Psychology, 11*, 502981.

Dehghansai, N., Pinder, R., & Baker, J. (2021). "Looking for a golden needle in the haystack": Perspectives on talent identification and development in Paralympic sport. *Frontiers in Sports and Active Living: Elite Sports and Performance Enhancement, 3*, 635977.

Dehghansai, N., Spedale, D., Wilson, M. J., & Baker, J. (2020b). Comparing developmental trajectories of elite able-bodied and wheelchair basketball players. *Adapted Physical Activity Quarterly, 37*(3), 338–348.

Douglas, S., Falcão, W. R., & Bloom, G. A. (2018). Career development and learning pathways of Paralympic coaches with a disability. *Adapted Physical Activity Quarterly, 35*(1), 93–110.

Dowling, M., Brown, P., Legg, D., & Grix, J. (2018). Deconstructing comparative sport policy analysis: Assumptions, challenges, and new directions. *International Journal of Sport Policy and Politics, 10*(4), 687–704.

Evans, M. B., Shirazipour, C. H., Allan, V., Zanhour, M., Sweet, S. N., Martin Ginis, K. A., & Latimer-Cheung, A. E. (2018). Integrating insights from the parasport community to understand optimal experiences: The Quality Parasport Participation Framework. *Psychology of Sport and Exercise, 37*, 79–90.

Gulbin, J. P., Croser, M. J., Morley, E. J., & Weissensteiner, J. R. (2013). An integrated framework for the optimisation of sport and athlete development: A practitioner approach. *Journal of Sports Sciences, 31*(12), 1319–1331.

Howe, P. & Jones, C. (2006). Classification of disabled athletes: (Dis)empowering the Paralympic practice community. *Sociology of Sport Journal, 23*, 29–46.

Hutzler, Y., Higgs, C., & Legg, D., (2016). Improving Paralympic development programs: Athlete and institutional pathways and organizational quality indicators. *Adapted Physical Activity Quarterly, 33*(4), 305–310.

Jeanes, R., Spaaij, R., Magee, J., Farquharson, K., Gorman, S., & Lusher, D. (2019). Developing participation opportunities for young people with disabilities? Policy enactment and social inclusion in Australian junior sport. *Sport in Society, 22*(6), 986–1004.

Kean, B., Gray, M., Verdonck, M., Burkett, B., & Oprescu, F. (2017). The impact of the environment on elite wheelchair basketball athletes: A cross-case comparison. *Qualitative Research in Sport, Exercise and Health, 9*(4), 485–498.

Legg, D. & Steadward, R. (2011). The Paralympic Games and 60 years of change (1948–2008): Unification and restructuring. In Jill M. Le Clair (Ed.) *Disability in the global sport arena: A sporting chance. Special edition of Sport in Society.* London: Taylor & Francis.

Lemez, S., Wattie, N., Dehghansai, N., & Baker, J. (2020). Developmental pathways of para athletes: Examining the sporting backgrounds of elite Canadian wheelchair basketball players. *Current Issues in Sport Science, 5*(2), 1–9.

Martin, J. J. (2015). Determinants of elite disability sport performance, *Kinesiology Review, 4*(1), 91–98.

May, C. (2020). Athlete Pathways and Development. Retrieved September 1, 2021 from https://www.clearinghouseforsport.gov.au/kb/athlete-pathways-and-development

Orr, K., Evans, M. B., Tamminen, K. A., & Arbour-Nicitopoulos, K. P. (2019). A scoping review of recreational sport programs for disabled emerging adults. *Research Quarterly for Exercise and Sport, 91*(1), 142–157.

Pankowiak, A. (2020). National Paralympic sport policy interventions and contexts influencing a country's Paralympic success: A realist-informed conceptual framework (Thesis). Retrieved from http://vuir.vu.edu.au/41801/. Available from EBSCOhost Victoria University Research Repository database.

Patatas, J. M. (2019). *Sports system and policy factors influencing athletic career pathways in Paralympic Sports* (published Doctoral dissertation, Vrije Universiteit Brussel). Brussels, Belgium: VUBPRESS.

Patatas, J. M., De Bosscher, V., Derom, I., & De Rycke, J. (2020). Managing parasport: An investigation of sport policy factors and stakeholders influencing para-athletes' career pathways. *Sport Management Review, 23*(5), 937–951.

Patatas, J. M., De Rycke, J., De Bosscher, V., & Kons, R. L. (2021). It's a long way to the top: Determinants of developmental pathways in Paralympic Sport. *Adapted Physical Activity Quarterly, 38*(4), 605–625.

Patatas, J. M., De Bosscher, V., Derom, I., & Winckler, C. (2022). Stakeholders' perceptions of athletic career pathways in Paralympic Sport: From participation to excellence. *Sport in Society, 25*(2), 299–320.

Pensgaard, A. M., & Sorensen, M. (2002). Empowerment through the sport context: A model to guide research for individuals with disability. *Adapted Physical Activity Quarterly, 19*(1), 48–67.

Poucher, Z. A., Sabiston, C. M., Cairney, J., Kerr, G., & Tamminen, K. A. (2021). *An examination of the prevalence of mental disorders among elite Canadian athletes in an Olympic (and pandemic) year* [Oral]. North American Society for the Psychology of Sport and Physical Activity, online.

Poucher, Z. A., Tamminen, K. A., Sabiston, C. M., Cairney, J., & Kerr, G. (2020). *Prevalence of common mental disorders among elite Canadian athletes* [Poster]. Sport Canada Research Initiative Conference, online.

Richardson, E. V., Smith, B., & Papathomas, A. (2017). Crossing boundaries: The perceived impact of disabled fitness instructors in the gym. *Psychology of Sport and Exercise, 29*, 84–92.

Rohwerder, B. (2018). *Disability stigma in developing countries. Knowledge Evidence and learning for development.* Retrieved September 10, 2021 from https://www.ids.ac.uk/publications/disability-stigma-in-developing-countries/

Seggie, J. (2012). Going for gold – More ability, less disability. *South African Medical Journal, 102*(11), 813.

South African Sport Association for the Physically Disabled (2021). *History.* Retrieved September 1, 2021 from https://www.sasapd.org.za/history/

Stone-MacDonald, A., & Butera, G. (2014). Cultural beliefs and attitudes about disability in East Africa. *Review of Disability Studies, 8*(1), 1–19.

Wareham, Y., Burkett, B., Innes, P., & Lovell, G. P. (2018). Coaches of elite athletes with disability: Senior sports administrators' reported factors affecting coaches' recruitment and retention. *Qualitative Research in Sport, Exercise and Health, 11*(3), 398–415.

Williams, G. (2021). Coaching on the talent pathway: The influence of developmental experiences on coaching [Oral]. QRSE Student Conference, online.

3

TOP-DOWN SYSTEMIC CHALLENGES TO CURRENT PARALYMPIC PATHWAYS

Jacqueline M. Patatas and Veerle De Bosscher
Practitioner Commentary: Andy Van Neutegem

Introduction

Sports offer an important platform for countries to gain international prestige and diplomatic recognition. Effective elite sport policy will influence the development of successful elite athlete pathways – which in turn, is vital for gaining a competitive international advantage (De Bosscher et al., 2015; Sotiriadou et al., 2008). Sports-related literature has increasingly examined and delineated the elements of non-disabledsports systems linked to the production of successful elite athletes (De Bosscher et al., 2015; Digel et al., 2006; Green & Houlihan, 2005; Houlihan & Green, 2008; Sotiriadou et al., 2008). Paralympic sport system and athletes with an impairment, in contrast, have been underexplored (Pankowiak, 2020; Patatas, 2019). In this chapter, we will attempt to address this issue by reviewing the wide range of factors that directly impact Paralympic pathways development from a sport policy perspective. In doing so, we will consider sport policies that explicitly target the development of Para sport athletes; through that, we use the sports policy literature as a guide to identify the policy-related challenges to current Paralympic pathways.

Para sport policies

In comparison to the extensive knowledge that has been produced regarding the delivery and implementation of non-disabled sport policies, Para sport-specific perspectives have lagged behind. Insights and recommendations on how sport policies embedded in the Para sport context can influence athlete development are sorely needed. As this chapter seeks to explore the top-down

DOI: 10.4324/9781003184430-3

approaches to current Paralympic pathways, it is important to understand how Para sport policies can be developed differently from policies in non-disabled sport. Another point to consider is how organisations communicate and facilitate resources that can have a great impact on the accessibility and availability of resources for optimal developmental environments for athletes. Consequently, policymakers' knowledge of Para sport influences the way the policy agenda that contours Paralympic pathways is developed and implemented (Patatas et al., 2020).

Grounded in the lens of disability studies, Patatas et al. (2020) suggested the classification system(s) used in Para sport add one more layer of complexity when addressing sport policies in the Para sport context. According to the authors, classification should be seen as a common factor that influences policy development and implementation. We can therefore assume that the trajectories of Para sport athletes through an athletic career pathway may vary according to the sport class to which an athlete is allocated. According to Patatas et al., (2022), impairment type(s) and classification could dictate the sports where athletes have a greater opportunity for development. Additionally, the transition out of the sport (e.g., involuntary retirement) is another example of how classification can influence Para athletes' trajectories (e.g., reclassification, changes in classification rules and regulations, ineligibility; Bundon et al., 2018). From a systemic perspective, instead of solely identifying talented athletes, nations may first identify which class within a sport would represent a higher likelihood of winning medals. Para athletes are then identified as having – or not having – talent according to this likelihood of future success; as a result, those considered 'talented' may receive more financial support throughout their careers. Put differently, the way classification operates and directs the top-down approaches in Para sport is simple: the factors of particular sport classes (for instance, few athletes competing in a class), a low technical level of athletes in a given class, or how the sports events are distributed and (not) included in the Paralympic Games programme can serve as critical parameters for policies towards talent identification (Patatas, 2019).

Sport policy and success

The state-of-the-art literature in the elite sport policy field (Bergsgard et al., 2007; Böhlke, 2007; De Bosscher et al., 2006, 2015; Digel et al., 2006; Green & Houlihan, 2005; Oakley & Green, 2001) has revealed several factors that can influence athlete development and, consequently, international sporting success. The general characteristics found in those studies reflect common key policy areas that are essential for developing and moving athletes along the pathway, in both Para sport and non-Para sport contexts (e.g., financial support, training facilities, coaching, talent identification, and post-career support; Patatas et al., 2020).

From the contemporary sport policy literature, one study in particular was beneficial for guiding this chapter, as it is one of the most comprehensive frameworks covering the policy-related factors considered necessary across the trajectory (from foundation to retirement) of athletic development (Hutzler et al., 2016; Patatas et al., 2020). The SPLISS framework (*Sport Policy Factors Leading to International Sporting Success*; De Bosscher et al., 2006, 2015) is based on an extensive review of the literature and reflects the necessary ingredients for developing sporting success. De Bosscher et al. (2006, 2015) offer a framework that aims to explain the relationship between elite sport policy and international sporting success. They base their views on two premises. The first is that sporting success can be developed. The second is that factors determinative of international success occur at three levels: macro (environment), meso (policy), and micro (talent). However, it is only at the meso level that success can be cultivated. The framework was firstly empirically tested in six countries (SPLISS 1.0; De Bosscher et al., 2006) and later further refined in a comparison of 15 countries (SPLISS 2.0; De Bosscher et al., 2015). The SPLISS framework consists of nine pillars (or sport policy dimensions) that influence international sporting success; it also specifies 31 sub-dimensions and 96 critical success factors as critical elements within pillars that are necessary to improve the elite sport success of a nation (De Bosscher et al., 2015). The nine sport policy dimensions derived from the SPLISS framework are *(1) financial support; (2) governance, organisation and structure of sport policies; (3) foundation and participation; (4) talent identification system and talent development; (5) athletic career support and post-career support; (6) training facilities; (7) coaching provision and coach development; (8) (inter)national competition; and (9) scientific research.*

In the following section, we review the systemic challenges currently existing in Paralympic pathways underpinned by the lens of the SPLISS framework (De Bosscher et al., 2006, 2015) (Figure 3.1).

Learning to see challenges as opportunities

Even though the SPLISS framework is built upon the non-disabled sport contexts, the studies from Patatas et al. (2018, 2020) contend that, in general, the policy dimensions noted within this framework are important and offer some critical elements that can serve as the best principles to the Para sport context. On that note, in addition to tailoring the policy agenda to adequately fit the specific needs of Para athletes, one should not overlook the essential characteristics that make Paralympic sport distinctive from its non-disabled counterpart (Dowling et al., 2018). Accordingly, Patatas et al. (2018)

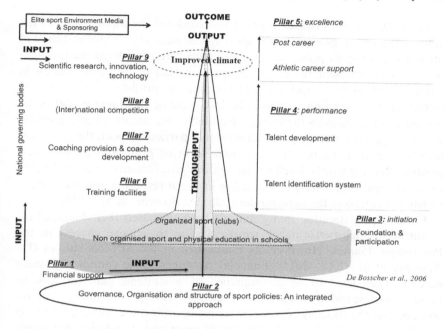

FIGURE 3.1   SPLISS model (Sport Policy factors Leading to International Sporting Success; De Bosscher et al., 2006)

explored how Paralympic stakeholders made meaning of the nine sport policy dimensions of the SPLISS framework (De Bosscher et al., 2006, 2015) as they would be applied to the Para sport context. Following that, Patatas et al. (2020) built upon the nine policy dimensions and critical success factors of SPLISS, and identified a range of elements that can be considered as Para sport-specific policy and organisational factors that facilitate the development of Paralympic pathways. Conceivably, these elements – taken together with the context in which Para sport operates – could assist in developing a framework that could advise sport policymakers on optimising their elite sport systems to achieve Paralympic success.

One of the insights that we expect to offer in this chapter is not that one should use the SPLISS framework (De Bosscher et al., 2006, 2015) as a blueprint for the Para sport system but, rather, stakeholders should further adopt an approach that embraces a combination of an existing model such as SPLISS, while considering the unique ingredients from the Para sport context, such as those outlined next.

Financial support

The pillars, or sport policy dimensions, of the SPLISS framework (De Bosscher et al., 2006, 2015) represent a logical model of *Inputs, Throughputs,*

Outputs, Outcome. Financial support is considered the input pillar, as the inflow of financial resources to the sport system allows the implementation of the other eight sport policy dimensions. Those are considered the through-puts as they represent the processes that can lead to increased success in international sports competitions. The output – or product – is the achieved results, that is, sporting success. The last stage of this logic model is the outcome, which assesses the impacts (results) of the success of elite sport on society in general, such as public interest in a particular sport, the growth in membership of a particular sport, and sense of pride and international prestige. In other words, it reflects the reasons governments invest in the elite sports system, particularly by inputting financial resources into the system, which will complete the logic model cycle (De Bosscher et al., 2015).

For the past decades, many nations have increased their financial investment in high-performance sports, aiming to achieve success in the Paralympic Games. However, as established in the SPLISS studies (De Bosscher et al., 2006, 2015), financial resources alone cannot guarantee success. They need to be accompanied by a strategic plan for how to manage and spend the resources efficiently. Though the amount of resources that the sport system possesses is important, the 'game changer' is usually the organisation and structure of sport and its relationship to society that enables efficient use of these resources (De Bosscher et al., 2015).

A common challenge faced by most sport organisations in the Paralympic context is the higher costs involved with Para sport participation (e.g., sport equipment such as wheelchairs, assistive devices such as prostheses, and the need for additional staff such as athlete guides for athletes with visual impairments; Patatas et al., 2018). A successful Para sport system should focus on bridging the gap between the resources spent with the high-performance and the Para sport grassroots system by building a broad base of sport participation. This may increase the chances of achieving success in the long term (Patatas et al., 2018).

Governance, organisation, and structure of sport policies

Well-structured and organised sport policies form the backbone of a successful sport system. Those require effective national coordination, long-term planning, clear communication, decision making, and collaboration with a wide range of stakeholders. However, there is no 'one-size-fits-all' formula about the best approach to developing and implementing elite sport policies and governance (De Bosscher et al., 2015). One significant difference between non-disabled and Para sport systems is related to governance. Unlike non-disabled sports that are organised by international sports federations, the Paralympic sport organisation umbrella is composed by:

International Federations (IF) in the four international structures: sport-specific and segregated, i.e., parasport-specific federations (e.g., wheelchair basketball [IWBF]); sport-specific and integrated, i.e., parasport as part of the able-bodied sport federation (e.g., wheelchair tennis [ITF]); impairment-specific and segregated, i.e., the International Organisations of Sport for the Disabled (IOSDs) (e.g., judo [IBSA]); and IPC sports, i.e., the IPC act as an International Federation (e.g., athletics, swimming). The IOSDs are vital organisations in the structure of Paralympic sports, which are independent organisations recognised by the IPC as the sole representatives of a specific impairment group. (Patatas, 2019, p. 44)

Because there are several organisations involved in Para sport governance, Para sport policies are organised on a vastly different basis when compared to non-disabled systems (Legg et al., 2003). This may represent a challenge for several sport systems, therefore, it is recommended that the organisation and structure of sport policies are developed coherently and holistically. Delineating the responsibilities of different agencies, ensuring effective communication between all stakeholders, and simplifying administration can maximise the chances of sporting success (De Bosscher et al., 2015; Oakley & Green, 2001). In addition, it is reasonable to recommend the inclusion of persons with impairments in the decision-making process as a means of further incorporating their own views on how sports organisations could better develop and implement policies to further contribute to efficiencies in Paralympic pathways (see 'Nothing about us, without us!'; Charlton, 1998).

Foundation and participation

Scholars in the field argue that it is necessary to create and implement sports policies for both high-performance and grassroots sports, as a broad participation pyramid is crucial in the pursuit of sporting success (De Bosscher et al., 2015). We can therefore assume that a broad base of participation can influence sporting success due to the continued supply of young talents to high-performance sport. The SPLISS framework uses three levels of analysis as a parameter to assess whether the sport's participation policy at the national level has an impact on the success of elite sport, namely: (a) opportunities for children to participate in sports at school (physical education or extracurricular activities); (b) existence of a generally high level of participation in sport in the country (sports culture); and (c) the existence of a national policy to promote the implementation of actions aimed at sports development for clubs and federations (De Bosscher et al., 2015). For Para sports, however, the big question revolves around where the person with an impairment will have access to Para sport (i.e., attraction to sport). For example, in non-disabled sport, children usually have several opportunities to have their first contact with sport within the school environment (Patatas et al., 2018). This may not be the reality for children with impairments, as they may not be inserted in an environment where the sport is provided for them at school, or because there are no qualified professionals to offer sports practice to children with impairments (Patatas et al., 2022). Consequently, the first contact with the sport, in this case, is dependent on some action outside the school, which can be in clubs or rehabilitation centres.

Talent identification and development

After entering the sports system, an important part of the transition process between the phases of an athletic career is to ensure that sport policies will be implemented so that young talents can be identified and developed (Radtke & Doll-Tepper, 2014). The constant search for success requires that the sport system not only allows a sustained level of performance in international competitions but is also concerned with the continuous development of talented athletes, in other words, the sustainability of the system (De Bosscher et al., 2008). Hence the importance of policies to inform the detection, selection, and promotion of sports talents who in the future will represent their country in major international competitions, such as the Paralympic Games and World Championships (Patatas et al., 2022). An important challenge to consider, however, is the fact that in the Paralympic context talent identification is limited by the smaller pool of athletes available for selection (Radtke & Doll-Tepper, 2014). This results in extra challenges for foundation programmes such as the 'Bridging the Gap' programme developed in Canada which aims to introduce people with impairments to wheelchair sport opportunities and to support ongoing physical activity. The limited pool of athletes at the grassroots level has impacted the systematic identification and development of the next generation of elite Para athletes. Finally, the Para sport system is a 'classification-oriented system' in terms of athlete identification and development (Patatas et al., 2020). The classification, therefore, may influence and dictate how a Para sport athlete is identified as a talent and, in later phases (i.e., leading towards elite) the type and amount of resources and supports that the athlete will receive (Patatas et al., 2022).

Athletic career and post-career support

In general, the development of an athletic career follows a standardised process in which after identifying the talent, there is usually a transition to the elite phase (or high-performance). This transition to elite can happen quickly in the path of a Paralympic athlete (Patatas et al., 2018, 2020, 2022). In this sense, Para sport athletes progress in the stages of development while still acquiring and improving their motor skills, accompanied by a set of demands and challenges for practice and competition (Patatas et al., 2020). According to De Bosscher et al. (2015), the focus of sport policies in this phase should be on achieving national and international sports success. In order to do so, the implementation of policies should aim not only to support athletes during their sports careers but also to establish ways for these athletes to be able to create opportunities for their lives post-sport career. However, this may represent a challenge for some sport systems that fail to recognise the need to holistically approach the development of sports policies and support for post-career (Patatas, 2019). It is necessary that strategic planning broadens its objectives to contemplate the retirement of athletes and their transition out of the sport (Patatas et al., 2022). This could be achieved by providing support for Para athletes who want to attain management roles or become coaches after retiring from their athletic career. According to Itoh et al. (2018), such policies remain rather scarce in the Paralympic movement.

(Accessible) training facilities

Sports facilities such as training centres can encourage the exchange of knowledge between sports. Infrastructure and equipment are important success factors in the process of enabling athletes to train in a relevant and high-quality sporting environment (De Bosscher et al., 2015). Consequently, training facilities are essential for the development of both non-disabled and Para sport athletes; however, modifications may be necessary to accommodate the accessibility needs of Para athletes (McPherson et al., 2017). Scholars agree that accessibility at training facilities has been an enduring challenge for Paralympic pathways and can directly hinder athletic development (Dehghansai et al., 2020; Jaarsma et al., 2014). The key policy action here is to ensure training facilities are accessible. Once these barriers are removed, sport participation may increase, resulting in a bigger pool of athletes moving along the pathways (Dehghansai et al., 2020). Brazil is a good example, as the country has demonstrated solid management of the Brazilian Paralympic Training Centre (one of the greatest legacies of the Rio 2016 Paralympic Games). The training centre covering 95 thousand square meters, has indoor and outdoor facilities that are fully accessible for training, competitions, and exchanges of athletes and teams. In addition, policies were created to promote Paralympic sport in Brazil and increase the inclusion of people with impairments in society (Patatas et al., 2021).

Coaching provision and development

Coaching provision is a policy factor strongly highlighted in the literature as needing further consideration when applied to the Para sport context. Several authors (Douglas et al., 2018; Huntley et al., 2019; Taylor et al., 2014; Townsend et al., 2018; Wareham et al., 2018) have pointed out that access to quality coaches possessing disability-specific knowledge is indispensable in developing Para sport athletes. On that note, Para sport coaches must be capable of considering the unique physiological challenges of each athlete (each often with his/her unique sets of impairments and with particular needs such as specialised sports equipment, prosthetics, and medications, as may directly impact training plans; Taylor et al., 2014). The studies from Patatas et al. (2020, 2022) indicate that promoting training and building capacity for coaches is the most influential sports policy factor throughout an athletic career pathway. In addition, the authors draw attention to the fact that coaches are the stakeholders most highly involved during most phases of athlete development. According to the critical success factors highlighted in the SPLISS framework, there are strong and significant correlations between the overall quality of training and capacity of coaches and sporting success (De Bosscher et al., 2015). This reinforces the need to provide inclusive policies and practices that support the training and qualification for coaches to gain disability-specific knowledge from the beginning of Para athletes' sporting careers (Patatas et al., 2020).

(Inter)national competitions

De Bosscher et al. (2015) theorised that one of the processes for achieving sporting success is in the ability of athletes to participate in international competitions and the organisation of national and international events in the country. For Paralympic pathways, participation in competition represents an important step towards talent identification and development (Patatas et al., 2022). Often, it is during participation in competitions that development coaches and officers recognise the 'talent' of Para athletes (Patatas et al., 2021). However, the organisation of competitions at the regional or national level can be a challenge due to the small pool of Para athletes with the same classification. In some cases, when the pool of athletes is not enough to provide the ideal competition experience, the common solution is to merge athletes with different classifications competing at the same event. However, this situation may not be ideal because it allows the athlete to experience a situation that is not 'real' compared to the international level, causing a less optimal environment for athletes to prepare themselves for international competitions (Patatas et al., 2022). As a result, the lack of regional or national competition opportunities can hinder Para sport athlete development (Patatas et al., 2020).

Scientific research

Scientific research on elite sport is one of the fastest-growing fields of interest in the past decade and is proving to be an increasingly important factor in the pursuit of sporting success. The nations with the best international performance generally make good investments in scientific research and innovation (De Bosscher et al., 2015). Even though there has been an increase in research addressing Paralympic sport, the area is still underdeveloped and lacking investments in several countries (Patatas et al., 2018). On the one hand, the uniqueness of Paralympic sport (e.g., idiosyncrasies of the Paralympic classification and its effects on athletes' performance, biomechanics and physiology, health issues and potential injuries, thermoregulation in athletes with spinal cord injuries, etc.) may create novel challenges for developing research in this vast area (Keogh, 2011). On the other hand, there are still many opportunities for research to contribute to our understanding of the determinants of optimal development of Paralympic pathways.

Conclusion

Taken together, the way Para sport policies are shaped and implemented requires a holistic, flexible, and context-specific approach. As emphasised by Houlihan (2005), considering the context is essential for effective sport policy, both in terms of development and implementation. In this sense, the contextual factors in a specific society or sport are crucial for analysing policy development, insofar as initial policy decisions can determine future policy choices (Houlihan & Green, 2009). To conclude, the investigation of central sport policy factors that contribute to the development of successful Paralympic pathways is a burgeoning area of research that needs to be further addressed. With this chapter, we hope to have opened the dialogue and offered primary insights and recommendations on how sport policies, as embedded in the Paralympic sport context, can impact Paralympic pathways development.

Practitioner commentary

The authors provide an excellent analysis of a Paralympic Pathway using the SPLISS model (Sport Policy Factors Leading to International Sporting Success; De Bosscher et al., 2006, 2015) as a lens to understand challenges, or opportunities related to Para sport pathways. It is rightly acknowledged that the model may not adequately account for the experience of Para athletes in their journey from playground to podium, or perhaps more accurately in many situations, from hospital bed to podium. Yet ironically the model is still used as a framework to explore what it takes to achieve

Paralympic podium success with modifications to the nine pillars reflecting the Para sport context. Perhaps, a better approach is to not start from a model based on 40 years of extensive research and including surveys involving athletes, coaches, and performance directors that undoubtedly have little or no experience with the Paralympic context. Why must our (re-) imagining of Paralympic success and facilitative policies start with a non-disabled perspective? Imagine a SPLISS model driven entirely from the Paralympic context using opinions from global leaders, athletes and coaches involved in Paralympic sport.

Of course, this is not to suggest similar SPLISS pillars would not also be identified for a Paralympic model of sport policy factors influencing international success. But the SPLISS pillars are based on 103 different critical success factors (CSFs) grouped thematically according to the different stages of athletic development. Given the differences between a non-disabled athlete and an athlete with an impairment, it is likely that a SPLISS equivalent model for elite Para sport would appear significantly different diagrammatically, and perhaps feature a re-ordering of what is considered an input, throughput, output, and outcome. Further, the weight of each pillar in terms of importance may also differ significantly in the Para athlete's journey.

The impact of classification on athletic development is perhaps the best example of the different pathway experienced by a Para athlete compared to a non-disabled athlete. The authors correctly point out its impact on shaping the trajectory towards a podium and potential for specific policies to manage its effect on athlete development. Classification has always been intended to facilitate participation and streamline performance opportunities for athletes having similar impairments. In many ways, classification is a pillar of a Para athlete pathway given its input role in determining the potential pathway trajectory, transfer within and between sports based on function, and the type of equipment, coaching and training, and competition experiences that may be available and required to sustain pathway progression.

Perhaps a missing sport policy dimension in SPLISS relevant to Paralympic sport is policy facilitation of an inclusive environment that supports the identification and development of a Paralympic athlete as well as their successful exit from an athletic career. Although, funding was determined in the SPLISS model to be a core input to successful nations coupled with system efficiency, an inclusive environment (which is more than just an accessible training facility) provides a safe environment for the athlete with an impairment to develop their unique identity as a Paralympic athlete, respected for their differences from non-disabled athletes. It is this input from the start that sets the stage for successful athlete development and the ability to navigate the fragility of classification and provide the identity anchor to successfully manage a successful transition out of sport into a society that sees the whole person rather than a 'disabled' one. Coaches who understand the unique identity of a Paralympic athlete and socialisation process of being born with or acquiring an impairment may be better equipped to facilitate a different journey for the Para sport athlete and yet still strive for the same goal of podium success as their non-disabled counterpart.

An inclusive environment may be consistent backdrop to any critical successful factors for Paralympic success. It permeates the Input, Throughput, Output, and Outcomes. Finally, models such as SPLISS often start with the end in mind which is often calculated using medal counts, and Top 8 finishes. A Paralympic pathway should reflect the Paralympic Movement in which the outcome is about celebrating diversity and showing that difference is a strength. The strength and value of a Paralympic pathway is not who the person is standing on the podium but rather who they have become many years later as members of our society.

References

Bergsgard, N. A., Houlihan, B., Mansget, P., Nodland, S. I., & Rommetveldt, H. (2007). *Sport policy: A comparative analysis of stability and change.* London, England: Elsevier.

Böhlke, N. (2007). New insights in the nature of best practice in elite sport system management – Exemplified with the organisation of coaches education. *New Studies in Athletics, 45*(3), 49–59.

Bundon, A., Ashfield, A., Smith, B., & Goosey-Tolfrey, V. L. (2018). Struggling to stay and struggling to leave: The experiences of elite para-athletes at the end of their sport careers. *Psychology of Sport & Exercise, 37*, 296–305.

Charlton, J. I. (1998). *Nothing about us without us: Disability oppression and empowerment.* Los Angeles, CA: University of California Press.

De Bosscher, V., Bingham, J., Shibli, S., van Bottenburg, M., & De Knop, P. (2008). *A global sporting arms race. An international comparative study on sports policy factors Leading to international sporting success.* Aachen, Germany: Meyer & Meyer.

De Bosscher, V., De Knop, P., van Bottenburg, M., & Shibli, S. (2006). A conceptual framework for analysing sports policy factors leading to international sporting success. *European Sport Management Quarterly, 6*, 185–215.

De Bosscher, V., Shibli, S., Westerbeek, H., & van Bottenburg, M. (2015). *Successful elite sport policies. An international comparison of the sports policy factors leading to international sporting success (SPLISS 2.0) in 15 nations.* Aachen, Germany: Meyer & Meyer.

Dehghansai, N., Spedale, D., Wilson, M. J., & Baker, J. (2020). Comparing developmental trajectories of elite able-bodied and wheelchair basketball players. *Adapted Physical Activity Quarterly, 37*(3), 338–348.

Digel, H., Burk, V., & Fahrner, M. (2006). *High-performance sport. An international comparison* (Vol. 9). Weilheim/Teck, Tubingen: Bräuer.

Douglas, S., Falcão, W. R., & Bloom, G. A. (2018). Career development and learning pathways of Paralympic coaches with a disability. *Adapted Physical Activity Quarterly*, *35*(1), 93–110.

Dowling, M., Legg, D., & Brown, P. (2018). Comparative sport policy analysis and Paralympic Sport. In I. Brittain & A. Beacom (Eds.) *Handbook of Paralympic Studies* (pp. 249–272). London, England: Palgrave Macmillan.

Green, M., & Houlihan, B. (2005). *Elite sport development: Policy learning and political priorities*. London, England: Routledge.

Houlihan, B. (2005). Public sector sport policy: Developing a framework for analysis. *International Review for the Sociology of Sport*, *40*(2), 163–185.

Houlihan, B., & Green, M. (2008). Comparative elite sport development. In B. Houlihan & M. Green (Eds.), *Comparative elite sport development: Systems, structures and public policy* (pp. 1–25). London, England: Butterworth-Heineman.

Houlihan, B., & Green, M. (2009). Modernization and sport: The reform of Sport Englnad and UK sport. *Public Administration*, *87*(3), 678–698.

Huntley, T. D., A. Whitehead, C. Cronin, C. Williams, G. Ryrie, & R. C. Townsend. (2019). *Pan-European Work Force Audit and Best Practice Case Study Report: The Experiences of Coaches in Paralympic and Disability Sport*. September 2019. Retrieved from: https://www.paracoach.eu/news/paracoach-releases-the-pan-european-workforce-audit-and-best-practice-case-study-report

Hutzler, Y., Higgs, C., & Legg, D. (2016). Improving Paralympic development programs: Athlete and institutional pathways and organizational quality indicators. *Adapted Physical Activity Quarterly*, *33*, 305–310.

Itoh, M., Hums, M. A., Arai, A., & Ogasawara, E. (2018). Realizing identity and overcoming barriers: Factors influencing female Japanese Paralympians to become coaches. *International Journal of Sport and Health Science*, *16*, 50–56.

Jaarsma, E., Dijkstra, P., Geertzen, J., & Dekker, R. (2014). Barriers to and facilitators of sports participation for people with physical disabilities: A systematic review. *Scandinavian Journal of Medicine & Science in Sports*, *24*, 871–881.

Keogh, J. W. (2011). Paralympic sport: An emerging area for research and consultancy in sports biomechanics. *Sports Biomechanics*, *10*(3), 234–253.

Legg, D., Wolff, E. A., & Hums, M. (2003). Relationships between international sport federations and international disability sport. CSSS research articles and reports, Paper 8.

McPherson, G., Misener, L., McGillivray, D., & Legg, D. (2017). Creating public value through parasport events. *Event Management*, *21*(2), 185–199.

Oakley, B., & Green, M. (2001). The production of Olympic champions: International perspectives on elite sport development system. *European Journal for Sport Management*, *8*, 83–105.

Pankowiak, A. (2020). *National Paralympic sport policy interventions and contexts influencing a country's Paralympic success: A realist-informed conceptual framework* (Doctoral dissertation, Victoria University).

Patatas, J. M. (2019). *Sports system and policy factors influencing athletic career pathways in Paralympic sports*. (Published Doctoral dissertation, Vrije Universiteit Brussel). Brussels, Belgium: VUBPRESS.

Patatas, J. M., De Bosscher, V., Derom, I., & De Rycke, J. (2020). Managing parasport: An investigation of sport policy factors and stakeholders influencing para-athletes' career pathways. *Sport Management Review*, *23*(5), 937–951.

Patatas, J. M., De Bosscher, V., Derom, I., & Winckler, C. (2022). Stakeholders' perceptions of athletic career pathways in Paralympic sport: From participation to excellence. *Sport in Society*, *25*(2), 299–320.

Patatas, J.M., De Bosscher, V., & Legg, D. (2018). Understanding parasport: An analysis of the differences between able-bodied and parasport from a sport policy perspective. *International Journal of Sport Policy and Politics*, *10*, 235–254.

Patatas, J. M., De Rycke, J., De Bosscher, V., & Kons, R. L. (2021). It's a long way to the top: Determinants of developmental pathways in Paralympic sport. *Adapted Physical Activity Quarterly*, *38*(4), 605–625.

Radtke, S., & Doll-Tepper, G. (2014). *A cross-cultural comparison of talent identification and development in Paralympic sports: Perceptions and opinions of athletes, coaches and officials.* Berlin: Freie Universität Berlin.

Sotiriadou, P., Shilbury, D., & Quick, S. (2008). The attraction, retention/transition, and nurturing process of sport development: Some Australian evidence. *Journal of Sport Management*, *22*, 247–272.

Taylor, S. L., Werthner, P., & Culver, D. (2014). A case study of a parasport coach and a life of learning. *International Sport Coaching Journal*, *1*, 127–138.

Townsend, R. C., Huntley, T. D., Cushion, C. J., & Fitzgerald, H. (2018). 'It's not about disability, I want to win as many medals as possible': The social construction of disability in high-performance coaching. *International Review for the Sociology of Sport*, *55*(3), 344–360.

Wareham, Y., Burkett, B., Innes, P., & Lovell, G. P. (2018). Coaches of elite athletes with disability: Senior sports administrators' reported factors affecting coaches' recruitment and retention. *Qualitative Research in Sport, Exercise and Health*, *11*(3), 398–415.

4

ATHLETE RECRUITMENT: PROMOTING INITIAL AND SUSTAINED ENGAGEMENT IN PARA SPORT

Joe Baker and Alia Mazhar
Practitioner Commentary: Michael Frogley

Introduction

Every athlete, from participants in local competitions to those attending Olympic and Paralympic Games, begins as a first-timer, in a new environment full of uncertainty, confusion and novelty. The pathway to this first-time experience is highly variable, and in Para sport settings, even more so. In this chapter, we focus on the issue of athlete recruitment. However, it is not possible to have a fulsome discussion of issues related to recruitment without framing this within the context of why successful recruitment is so important. Moreover, recruitment is only the first step in what, ideally, will become a long-term engagement in sport participation. As a result, we will discuss the range of social and cultural factors affecting the developmental landscape for athletes in Para sport.

At its most basic, recruitment refers to the explicit process of identifying, attracting, selecting, and onboarding athletes into a sporting program. This could be a program related to recreational engagement for the purposes of increased health, wellness, and functioning, or it could be a program more focused on high-performance outcomes. Regardless, the focus is on increasing the number of individuals *at the entry point* of the program (e.g., local recreation programs attracting new participants or a high-performance program looking for new athletes). Although the notion of athlete recruitment has not been widely explored in sport science (despite being similar to notions of 'talent detection' – see below) it is a key topic in human resources research (Newell, 2005; Roberts, 1997). In this context, recruitment is different from just increasing participation numbers. It relates to the active engagement of the 'right type' of individuals best suited

DOI: 10.4324/9781003184430-4

for available programs and the rejection of those who are unsuited. From this perspective, the intention is to improve system efficiency, particularly as it relates to the use of resources (Newell, 2005). This concern is shared with many practitioners working in Para sport settings due to the often-limited resources (e.g., athletes, funding, competition opportunities) in these systems (Dehghansai et al., 2020). That said, recruitment in Para sport is more difficult simply because the issues affecting system efficiency are more complex.

The recruitment process

Let's begin with an understanding of the process of recruitment. Ultimately, it is not enough to simply provide more and varied opportunities; an inappropriate initial engagement in Para sport (e.g., lack of success, low enjoyment) can have lasting effects. Given the importance of retaining athletes in Para sport, it is critical to promote continued engagement through the 'right type' of recruitment initiatives. In Figure 4.1, we provide a chain of decision-making that leads to a successful recruitment experience. This process is expanded from simply getting athletes 'through the door' and focuses on the quality of the recruitment experience as it relates to continued re-engagement in the sport. Below we consider each step in this decision-making process and explore how/where recruitment strategies may be effective.

Intention to participate

Most models of human behaviour recognize 'action' starts with an intention to 'do' something. However, intention results from attitudes and beliefs about the behaviour in question. As a result, an individual's intentions are influenced by broader factors related to their developmental milieu. For instance, in the well-known 'Theory of Planned Behaviour' (see Ajzen, 1991, but also Mummery & Wankel, 1999 for an application to training adherence in sport), intentions are influenced by attitudes individuals have about the behaviour (e.g., do I see this behaviour as positive or negative?), subjective norms regarding how others think about the behaviour (e.g., is participation valued by my peers?), and the degree to which the individual has control over the behaviour (e.g., how difficult would it be to participate?).

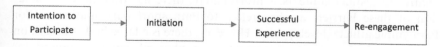

FIGURE 4.1   The process of successful initial engagement

Initiation

Once intentions are met, the likelihood of initiating the behaviour increases. The process of changing intentions into initiation is not straightforward and deterministic. Considerable research effort has been focused on what is called the 'intention-behaviour gap' (i.e., the failure to change intentions into actions, see Rhodes & de Bruijn, 2013). Furthermore, initiation takes place in a broader context of interests, motives and goals that affect how the initial participation experience is perceived and what it means for further engagement.

Successful experience

The factors influencing how current and future athletes define success may, at first, appear to be as varied as the athletes participating in the programs. However, evidence from motivation research suggests humans are similar in what drives their behaviour. Self-Determination Theory, for example, describes motivation as being relative to three fundamental and basic needs: the need for autonomy (i.e., feelings of personal control) the need for relatedness (i.e., feelings of social connection) and the need to feel competence (i.e., feelings of mastery or skill).

Re-engagement

As suggested above, continued patterns of behaviour such as sport training can be predicted by the degree to which basic needs and desires are met. Re-engagement can be measured in several ways, ranging from simple records of participation to more elaborate tracking of effort, enjoyment, and satisfaction across a program. In athlete development, re-engagement is the key mechanism promoting persistence in training, which leads to better learning outcomes, superior adaptations and eventually higher performance.

Barriers to recruitment in Para sport

In the next section we explore the range of factors affecting the recruitment of athletes into Para sport. These barriers may stem from social and cultural factors, thereby having more general effects, or they might be specific to the type of sport program being considered, having effects that are more relative to distinct contexts. Unfortunately, there has been little examination of these barriers as they relate to Para sport participation and/or Paralympic athlete development. However, there is a large body of work on barriers and obstacles to participation in physical activity amongst individuals with impairments (Martin Ginis et al., 2016). Since there is an obvious connection between these literatures ('sports' is a form of physical activity, after all), we will lay a broad foundation for the discussion, but emphasize that the extent to which these findings relate to high-performance athlete development requires considerable examination.

General barriers: Availability and accessibility

The most widely examined general barriers to participation relate to issues of availability and accessibility. Availability relates to the presence of resources. For instance, geographical location can impact the number of and type of facilities easily accessible to athletes with an impairment (Stephens et al., 2012). Depending on the type and severity of their impairment, Para sport athletes attempting to access facilities at a greater distance from their home face the barrier of transportation, which is not always reliable (Bragaru et al., 2013). Moreover, athletes with an impairment may be affected by time constraints that are different from their non-disabled counterparts (e.g., regular medical appointments) and these constraints may decrease the amount of time they can commit to sport (Aytur et al., 2018; Bragaru et al., 2013).

Accessibility, on the other hand, relates to the ability to utilize a resource. For example, cost is often identified as a barrier to Para sport participation. Stephens et al. (2012) found that cost related to equipment, training, competition, and travelling impacted Para athletes' participation. While there are some supports available to provide financial aid to Para athletes, this information is often obscure and is not easily accessed (McLoughlin et al., 2017). Furthermore, high-performance sporting organizations have finite funds to recruit and develop athletes, and therefore, typically prioritize those with the greatest potential for the world championship or Paralympic success. As a result of financial constraints on the side of Para sport organizations, athletes may not be recruited despite having the drive, motivation, and commitment to the sport (Dehghansai et al., 2021).

Research has emphasized the role environmental barriers can have on physical activity participation among individuals with an impairment. In some cases, for example, facilities are not wholly accessible. They may not have ramps or accessible changerooms, lack room to accommodate wheelchairs, and/or do not have adaptive equipment, all of which act as barriers to participation (Martin, 2013). Within the sports context, Stephens et al. (2012) found that facilities were generally not adapted to suit the needs of athletes with lower limb deficiencies. While these barriers persist across an athlete's development, they are particularly salient in deterring individuals from initial participation.

Notably, unlike in non-disabled sport where initial sport engagement usually begins in childhood, athletes with an impairment can enter sport from a range of developmental and maturational stages (e.g., athletes with newly acquired impairments due to trauma or disease), and 'accessibility' may mean different things to athletes at different stages of development (Dehghansai et al., 2022). Moreover, in some cases due to the nature of the athlete's impairment, support from non-disabled individuals may be required for initial or continued participation in sport. Despite this need, some Para athletes dislike seeking support from others in order to participate (Bragaru et al., 2013). Complicating things further, those providing support (e.g., parents and caregivers) may have challenges; for example, they may struggle with allocating adequate time for both their child with an impairment and children without impairments (Jaarsma et al., 2014). These barriers for athletes and their caregivers need to be addressed in order to transform intention to initiation and then to sustained engagement.

General barriers: Social stereotypes and preconceptions

Research indicates negative societal attitudes towards disability can negatively impact participation in physical activity among individuals with impairments (Levins et al., 2004). For example, individuals with an impairment who are physically inactive are perceived in a negative light when compared to their active counterparts (Kittson et al., 2013), which may make it more difficult to move from intention and interest into initiation and engagement. Iwuka and colleagues (2017) argued stigmatization of individuals with impairments negatively impact sports participation. For example, athletes with spinal cord injuries (Stephens et al., 2012) and lower limb amputees (Bragaru et al., 2013) have reported feeling patronized by the public, which acted as an additional barrier to continued sport engagement.

Specific barriers: Classification

Paralympic sports align with, and are governed by, codes set out by the International Paralympic Committee (IPC). The IPC sets the standards for which disability classifications can participate in major competitions and determines the measurement criteria for deciding how athletes are classified. As a result, athlete recruitment into high-performance systems can be influenced by the IPC's classification structure. For instance, recruitment into a Paralympic system might be strategically driven by an athlete's current level of performance *and* level of classification (sometimes current performance is not even considered; Dehghansai et al., 2021), which gives them a high probability of medalling at a Paralympics or World Championships (see Chapter 6, for an in-depth overview of classification's impact on talent identification and selection). Alternately, in some team sports the rules dictate the amount and type of classification allowed during competition. For instance, in wheelchair basketball, players are classified on a scale from 1.0 to 4.5 based on their level of physical function (1.0 is the lowest score) and a team can only have a total of 14.0 points among the five players on the court at any given time. As a result, coaches will use players' classifications strategically in building their team to maximize likelihood of success. All this to say, the unfortunate reality is that an athlete's motivation and desire to participate is only one element in the recipe for sporting success.

Specific barrier: Resourcing

As noted earlier, opportunities for participation are constrained by resourcing and this element is notoriously lower in Para sport programs compared to non-disabled sport contexts. The type of resourcing varies across the athlete development pathway. For instance, a local clubs'/programs' existence may depend on the number of participants they are able to bring into the program each season. Greater resourcing for this type of program may take the form of reduced fees that allow greater access to facilities, and/or hiring of qualified instructors so that programs are led by those knowledgeable about the specific needs of athletes with an impairment. In elite, high-performance programs, by way of comparison, funding comes almost entirely through government sponsorship, and increased resourcing in this program may involve greater support for athletes so they can meet day-to-day needs and/or opportunities to travel for competition and training. Ultimately, resourcing affects recruitment at each stage of the pathway by determining the amount and type of participation initiatives that are available.

Interaction of factors

Increasing the complexity of athlete recruitment in Para sport is recognition that these barriers, and other factors affecting athlete development function as part of a dynamic and inter-connected system. In Para sport settings, recruitment may be more appropriately positioned from the perspective of 'what does the system need currently?' and 'what will the system need in the future?'. These questions, obviously inter-connected, will help administrators, policymakers and coaches determine the most suitable approaches for driving recruitment into their program. In 2020, Dehghansai and colleagues developed a systems-based framework for exploring athlete development in Para sport (see Figure 4.2). This new framework was grounded in Newell's (1986) constraints-based model but expanded to capture the complexity of development in Para sport contexts. In this model, elements of

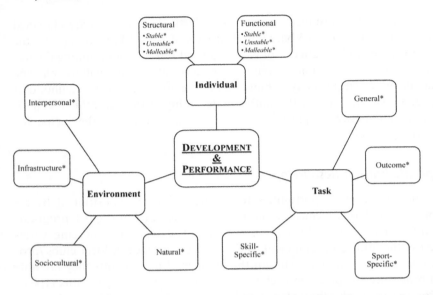

FIGURE 4.2 Dehghansai et al.'s (2020) modification of Newell's constraints-led model for Para sport

athlete development are related to interactions between the performer, their developmental and competition environments, and the features of the task.

Performer constraints

In their expanded framework, Dehghansai et al. (2020) created sub-categories of performer constraints, several of which are relevant to discussions of recruitment. For instance, the authors explored the differences between structural (i.e., body structure) and functional (behaviour) constraints, and whether the influence of these factors was stable or malleable over time. From a recruitment perspective, we are interested in how these constraints affect a) an individual's initial interest in Para sport (e.g., what promoted their interest?) and b) their initial level of success in that sport (e.g., did they enjoy it and are they more likely to return?).

Environment constraints

These elements relate to environmental factors that can affect development and performance. In Figure 4.2, this broad category is divided into four sub-categories to capture the nuances of how the environment can affect athlete development. This includes natural (e.g., climate, geography), infrastructure (e.g., accessibility and availability), sociocultural (e.g., policies, social beliefs and values), and interpersonal variables (e.g., social support and influential others).

Task constraints

Task constraints relate to explicit and implied rules of participation, goals of the sport and so on. In the model by Dehghansai et al. (2020), this category was sub-divided into *general task constraints* (e.g., primary elements necessary for participation such as the ability to push a wheelchair or grip/swing a racquet), *outcome task constraints* (elements related to the outcome of the task such as win/loss or points scored), *sport-specific task constraints* (elements such as rules, parameters, and equipment within the sport that provide the competition structure) and *skill-specific task constraints* (elements related to an individual's ability to adopt and excel in a specific task).

Although we have presented these factors as separate, it is important readers be reminded that the *interactions between the categories* are at the heart of Newell's approach and this proposed framework. Individual constraints, such as an athlete's functional capability to execute an overhand serve in wheelchair tennis, is directly related to how important the execution of this task constraint is to successful performance. In turn, these factors interact with a) the capacity of the training environment to provide the support for the athlete to acquire this skill (e.g., do the coaches have the skill to do this?) and b) the cost of this provision (e.g., does the system have the resources to make this feasible?).

Paralympian 'search' events: Are they an effective recruitment initiative?

The use of 'search' events has proliferated in many sporting nations, including Canada's Paralympian Search (Canadian Paralympic Committee, n.d.), UK Sport's fromhome2thegames (UK Sport, n.d.) and Australia's Talent 4 Tokyo (Paralympics Australia, n.d.). Generally, search events are intended to provide recruitment opportunities for sports to access community-based athletes currently outside the high-performance system. While the specific tests used during the events varies between countries, the objective is largely the same – to have athletes demonstrate their potential for success at the elite level. However, there has been very little exploration of these types of initiatives to assess their cost or benefits.

One exception is Dehghansai and Baker's (2020) descriptive examination of participants who attended 10 search events held in Canada between 2016 and 2018. The purpose of these events was to increase awareness, attract new athletes, and provide opportunities for experienced athletes to transfer between sports. Results indicated most of the participants at the events were male, young adults, and typically from the area close to where the search event took place. Interestingly, the study indicated these types of search events are generally effective at attracting athletes with a broad range of impairments and from a broad age range, but are generally already engaged in the sport system to some extent. As a result, this initial study suggests these types of events are not very effective at attracting new participants (i.e., non-athletes) to Para sport.

It's difficult to make any conclusions about the viability of these types of events given the sparse research in this area. The Dehghansai and Baker study suggests some value for identifying athletes who may already be participating at local or recreational levels but have not been identified by high-performance programs, but also suggests these events are less effective for driving new engagement initiatives. However, replication and extension of this work in other countries and in search programs with different objectives will be useful for determining the ultimate value of search programs for improving Para sport recruitment.

Recommendations for improving recruitment

Based on the challenges outlined above, in the next section we outline recommendations for improving recruitment for stakeholders in this area.

Recommendation 1: Build stronger links between levels of sport engagement

As a result of these obstacles to initial participation, many sports struggle to attain sufficient participants to provide programming in the first place. Thus, recruitment to drive participation numbers in a local program to sustain investment in the program over time is different from the type of recruitment necessary for high-performance sport programs, where participation may be more tightly controlled and regulated. However, these elements of the program are related, and engagement at all levels of Para sport would undoubtedly drive increasing numbers of participants into upper levels of skill and performance. Practitioners and stakeholders should make links between levels of sport engagement as strong and clear as possible.

Recommendation 2: Improve current initiatives

Most practitioners working in Para sport are aware of the limitations of current recruitment initiatives and are working hard to improve them. For instance, after the research by Dehghansai and Baker's (2020) Paralympian

Search events, the Canadian Paralympic Committee created initiatives directly focused on attracting and recruiting female athletes, since results suggested this was an under-served group in prior search events. Continued evaluation of recruitment initiatives and policies would undoubtedly identify other areas for improvement. Similarly, expanding initiatives to other, related fields (e.g., recruiting physiotherapists and physicians to introduce sport as a treatment modality for individuals with new or existing impairments; Douglas et al., 2018) may provide greater reach than existing approaches.

Recommendation 3: Balance needs and resources

In most Para sport contexts, it is important to recognize and acknowledge recruitment is a balance between individual needs and system resources. A greater understanding of individual behaviour (e.g., improving intentions and attitudes about participation) will only be helpful if there are resources in the system to promote this engagement. For example, individuals who may be well motivated and capable of being part of a national team for a given sport will ultimately be limited by the extent to which opportunities for that sport exist in their local area, and awareness of this local program within the structure of the high-performance athlete development system. To put it more bluntly, a person with an impairment with the potential to become the greatest Paralympic athlete in the world could be living in a small rural town at this moment, but the likelihood that they would ever have the opportunities for participation, and be detected/selected by a high-performance development program is minimal. Those working in Para sport need to be honest and transparent about limitations in their system since this awareness is necessary for improvement.

Recommendation 4: Recognize the varying pathways to success

A key difficulty faced by those working in Para sport settings is that athletes who enter the sport after an acquired injury can do so at any point in their development. For instance, Canadian Paralympian Sylvie Morel competed in wheelchair fencing at the recent Tokyo Paralympic Games at the age of 64, and did not start Paralympic competition (in Sydney 2000 Paralympic Games) until she was in her mid-40s. Contrasting that with Canada's youngest Paralympian at the same event, 17-year-old swimmer Nicholas Bennett, highlights the considerable range of 'developmental nuance' that needs to be considered when trying to understand how athletes find their way into Para sport (Dehghansai et al., 2021b).

Recommendation 5: Optimize the use of limited resources

Given the limited opportunities for Para sport, and the recognition that athlete recruitment into many sports is less than optimal, a better use of resources may come from a shared resource model. A model that focuses more broadly on general elements of participation across categories of sports, particularly during early development, may be helpful for making strained resources go further. For instance, a general program focused on improving movement quality and use of related equipment through participation in a broad range of wheelchair sports could be beneficial for athletes who might eventually move into high-performance programs (e.g., wheelchair basketball, wheelchair rugby, wheelchair tennis), while providing high-quality physical activity experiences for anyone who uses a wheelchair. Moreover, this type of general program has the potential to increase awareness of Para sports that are less well known (e.g., wheelchair softball or wheelchair soccer).

Improving recruitment: Where to focus and why

Based on the recommendations presented above, let's revisit the simple decision-making process originally presented in Figure 4.1. In Figure 4.3, this cognitive chain of events is expanded to reflect many of the recommendations in this chapter and provides a model for helping practitioners looking to design initiatives in this area.

Improving intentions

As noted, an individual's intentions are driven by broad psychosocial factors related to attitudes, norms, and control. For instance, they may be affected implicitly, such as when a society changes its valuation of individuals with impairments, thereby opening up social avenues (including sport) that may have been more difficult to access before these changes. Alternately, intentions may be changed using more explicit means. This approach is commonly reflected in 'talent detection' approaches, which broadly refer to the 'discovery of potential performers who are currently not involved in the sport in question' (Mohamed et al., 2009, p. 257). In this approach, potential athletes (e.g., females or athletes with a specific type of impairment) are targeted explicitly by providing opportunities that are not currently available (thereby improving elements of 'control') and emphasizing ways potential athletes can see themselves as elite-level performers (thereby emphasizing elements of 'relatedness' and 'competence'). Ideally, a mix of implicit and explicit approaches would be developed; although it is likely explicit approaches are quicker and easier to implement.

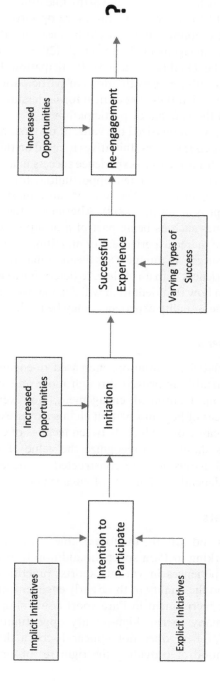

FIGURE 4.3 Integrating initiatives to increase the likelihood of successful initial engagement in Para sport

Increasing initiation and success

Bridging the intention-behaviour gap is a worthwhile outcome in itself, and future initiatives should focus on providing more opportunities for participation; however, these opportunities would be best served by increasing the quality of athletes' engagement. Evans et al. (2018; and Chapter 7 in this text) developed the Quality Parasport Participation Framework to emphasize participants' subjective evaluations of participation experiences, based on robust evidence that these are critical for understanding long-term engagement as well as the benefits of participation.

In an earlier section, we emphasized the value of understanding the variation in how individuals define success. Initiatives focused on this would ensure there are opportunities for athletes to experience success in a variety of ways. These may include performance-related opportunities for ego satisfaction (e.g., winning a match against a competitor) or more mastery-related outcomes (e.g., seeing improvement in a skill). Alternately, they may focus on socially related outcomes such as being part of a group that provides connection, enjoyment, and shared experience. For practitioners, recognizing that individuals will define success in unique ways means it may not be possible, at least during early experiences with an athlete, to determine a) how they define it at that moment or b) how that definition will change over time. Therefore, providing a range of high-quality experiences may be the best approach.

Promoting re-engagement

Like the initiatives related to initiation, increased re-engagement in Para sport could be most readily improved through more and better opportunities for participation. Continued engagement, however, requires recognition of the nuances of how motivation changes over extended periods of time. Moreover, because of the links between feelings of competence and motivation, initiatives should also recognize the value of managing how opportunities for skill acquisition are constructed for developing athletes since these are not independent elements of engagement and development.

Concluding thoughts

Athlete recruitment is and will, for the foreseeable future, remain a central concern for those working in Para sport. In addition to providing opportunities for initial experiences in various sports, practitioners should be encouraged to focus on the quality of these early engagements. Collectively, initiatives to improve recruitment in Para sport could simply be summarized as 'provide as many varied, high-quality opportunities as possible, as often as possible'. There does not appear to be a downside to this approach. The likelihood of providing the right set of circumstances for high-performance athlete development is increased *and* participants take with them an experience that is high in quality, satisfaction of their basic needs, and an increased likelihood of remaining a fan and supporter of Para sport. Recruitment of these latter individuals is also sorely needed for a sustainable and vibrant Para sport system.

Practitioner commentary

Several years ago, I returned from a Research 1 institution in the United States to start Wheelchair Basketball Canada's National Academy. From this background, I saw the value of research in sport and especially research in Para sport. One of the first researchers I met was Dr. Joe Baker. I saw how valuable his research was and the impact it could have. This most recent chapter will be no less impactful.

It is generally agreed that increasing athlete pool size is a major gap in Paralympic sport, with few exceptions, this is a focus in every Paralympic sport in every country around the world. While many programs try and grow their numbers, the effort is done without fully understanding the many variables that impact successful recruitment to a sport. The initial interaction an athlete has with a sport, directly and indirectly, can significantly impact whether they begin a journey in that sport. I can speak to that with first-hand knowledge having chosen not to play wheelchair basketball for two years after my initial experience in the sport.

Baker and Mazhar do an outstanding job at breaking down the system of recruitment and initial engagement so that we can understand more of the variables that impact these first two steps in an athlete's pathway. Too often, sport organizations simplify 'increasing numbers' to doing more demonstration programs or visiting more rehabilitation centers.

First, initial recruitment is more than just running a program. As the authors point out, first experiences have to contain a one-on-one interaction with the participants, the process must be easy to follow, and there needs to be an element of successful task execution for participants to be engaged.

Second, one of the great mistakes that is made in Para sport is retention, and this is rarely addressed. The authors point to the link between initial exposure and 're-engagement'. Without a pathway that is appropriately designed, there is likely to be a discrepancy between the skills athletes are taught and the skills necessary to develop and be successful in their sport.

I hope that as people read this chapter, they take the time to reflect and examine their recruitment programs with a critical eye to refining them and ensuring that all the variables the authors point to are present. If all these variables are not present and addressed, we will see recruitment programs that fall short, and we will see sports that continue to struggle with small athlete pools.

References

Ajzen, I. (1991). The theory of planned behavior. *Organizational Behavior and Human Decision Processes, 50*(2), 179–211.

Aytur, S., Craig, P. J., Frye, M., Bonica, M., Rainer, S., Hapke, L., & McGilvray, M. (2018). Through the lens of a camera: Exploring the meaning of competitive sport participation among youth athletes with disabilities. *Therapeutic Recreation Journal, 52*(2), 95–125.

Bragaru, M., van Wilgen, C. P., Geertzen, J. H. B., Ruijs, S. G. J. B., Dijkstra, P. U., & Dekker, R. (2013). Barriers and facilitators of participation in sports: A qualitative study on Dutch individuals with lower limb amputation. *PLoS ONE, 8*(3), e59881.

Canadian Paralympic Committee (n.d.). *Paralympian search.* Retrieved November 30, 2021 from https://paralympic.ca/paralympian-search

Dehghansai, N. & Baker, J. (2020). Searching for Paralympians: Characteristics of participants attending 'search' events. *Adapted Physical Activity Quarterly, 37*(1), 129–138.

Dehghansai, N., Lemez, S., Wattie, N., Pinder, R. & Baker, J. (2020). Understanding the development of elite parasport athletes using a constraints-led approach: Considerations for coaches and practitioners. *Frontiers in Psychology: Performance Science, 11*, 502981.

Dehghansai, N., Pinder, R. & Baker, J. (2021). "Looking for a golden needle in the haystack": Perspectives on talent identification and development in Paralympic sport. *Frontiers in Sports and Active Living: Elite Sports and Performance Enhancement, 3*, 635977.

Dehghansai, N., Pinder, R., & Baker, J. (2022). Pathways in Paralympic sport: An in-depth analysis of athletes' developmental trajectories and training histories. *Adapted Physical Activity Quarterly, 39*(1), 37–85.

Douglas, S., Falcão, W. R., & Bloom, G. A. (2018). Career development and learning pathways of paralympic coaches with a disability. *Adapted Physical Activity Quarterly, 35*(1), 93–110.

Evans, M. B., Shirazipour, C. H., Allan, V., Zanhour, M., Sweet, S. N., Ginis, K. A. M., & Latimer-Cheung, A. E. (2018). Integrating insights from the parasport community to understand optimal experiences: The Quality Parasport Participation Framework. *Psychology of Sport and Exercise, 37*, 79–90.

Ikwuka, F. N., Adeyemi., O. E., & Olaoye, A. K. (2017). Social and psychological determinants of sports participation among athletes with special needs in Abuja. *Benchmark Journals, 7*(2), 38–49.

Jaarsma, E. A., Dijkstra, P. U., Geertzen, J. H. B., & Dekker, R. (2014). Barriers to and facilitators of sports participation for people with physical disabilities: A systematic review. *Scandinavian Journal of Medicine and Science in Sports, 24*(6), 871–881.

Kittson, K., Gainforth, H., Edwards., J, Bolkowy, R., & Latimer-Cheung, A. (2013). The effect of video observation on warmth and competence ratings of individuals with a disability. *Psychology of Sport and Exercise, 14*, 847–851.

Levins, S., Redenbach, D., & Dyck, I. (2004). Individual and societal influences on participation in physical activity following spinal cord injury: A qualitative study. *Physical Therapy & Rehabilitation Journal, 84*(6), 496–509.

Martin, J. (2013). Benefits and barriers to physical activity for individuals with disabilities: A social-relational model of disability perspective. *Disability and Rehabilitation, 35*(24), 2030–2037.

Martin Ginis, K. A., Ma, J. K., Latimer-Cheung, A. E., & Rimmer, J. H. (2016). A systematic review of review articles addressing factors related to physical activity participation among children and adults with physical disabilities. *Health Psychology Review, 10*(4), 478–494.

McLoughlin, G., Fecske, C. W., Castaneda, Y., Gwin, C., & Graber, K. (2017). Sport participation for elite athletes with physical disabilities: Motivations, barriers, and facilitators. *Adapted Physical Activity Quarterly, 34*(4), 421–441.

Mohamed, H., Vaeyens, R., Matthys, S., Multael, M., Lefevre, J., Lenoir, M., & Philippaerts, R. (2009). Anthropometric and performance measures for the development of a talent detection and identification model in youth handball. *Journal of Sports Sciences, 27*(3), 257–266.

Mummery, W. K., & Wankel, L. M. (1999). Training adherence in adolescent competitive swimmers: An application of the theory of planned behavior. *Journal of Sport and Exercise Psychology, 21*(4), 313–328.

Newell, K. (1986). Constraints on the development of coordination. In M.W. Wade (Ed.) *Motor development in children: Aspects of coordination and control* (pp. 341–361). Martin Nijhoff.

Newell, S. (2005). Recruitment and selection. In S. Bach (Ed.) *Managing human resources: Personnel management in transition* (pp. 115–147). Blackwell.

Paralympics Australia (n.d.). *Targeting talent for Tokyo 2020.* Retrieved November 30, 2021 from https://www.paralympic.org.au/2016/03/talent-for-tokyo

Rhodes, R. E., & de Bruijn, G. J. (2013). How big is the physical activity intention–behaviour gap? A meta-analysis using the action control framework. *British Journal of Health Psychology, 18*(2), 296–309.

Roberts, G. (1997). *Recruitment and selection.* CIPD publishing.

Stephens, C., Neil, R., & Smith, P. (2012). The perceived benefits and barriers of sport in spinal cord injured individuals: A qualitative study. *Disability and Rehabilitation, 34*(24), 2061–2070.

UK Sport (n.d.). *Talent ID.* Retrieved November 30, 2021 from https://www.uksport.gov.uk/our-work/talent-id

5

UNDERSTANDING THE COMPLEXITY OF ATHLETE SELECTION IN PARALYMPIC SPORT

Nick Wattie and Nima Dehghansai
Commentary: Chris Wagg

The selection or non-selection of athletes is central to most levels of sport. Embedded in youth sports as try-outs, while at development and high-performance levels, the scouting mechanism is utilized by organizations (e.g., university programs, national sport organizations, professional sports teams, etc.) to select athletes. These selections essentially involve predictions about the short- and long-term potential of athletes. However, while ubiquitous, athlete selection is far from a homogenous process. Even within a single sport and league, decision-makers may take different approaches (e.g., the refutation or support of analytics: Gerrard, 2017). In comparison to non-disabled sports, there are unique and common challenges to decision-making to athlete selection in Para sport.

Definitions of talent vary greatly (see Baker & Wattie, 2018; Baker et al., 2019; Collins et al., 2019). Generally, however, talent refers to some characteristic that predicts future success. Some scholars have stipulated that talent is at least partially genetic in origin and therefore innate while others do not (Baker & Wattie, 2018; Howe et al., 1998). Many in the sport industry (e.g., researchers, coaches, scouts, announcers) find it exceptionally difficult to describe *what* talent is, relying on vague descriptors such as 'gifts' and assertions that they 'know it when they see it'. Indeed, academic descriptions of the properties of talent (see Baker & Wattie, 2018; Baker et al., 2019; Howe et al., 1998) do not provide a tangible sense of *what* to look for, beyond the assertion that this potential is multidimensional (e.g., physiological, anthropometric, psychological, cognitive). Regardless of how talent is defined or conceptualized, if 'talented' athletes can be identified reliably, resource allocation to optimize athlete development can be more efficient and effective. This is a pressing issue considering the finite resources that stakeholders

DOI: 10.4324/9781003184430-5

have to support athletes' development, particularly in Para sport. Furthermore, if talent can be identified accurately and reliably, it can reduce the occurrence of false positives and negatives, thereby further increasing the impact of these finite resources. However, because talent selection implies athletes are *only* selected for reasons to do with talent, which may not always be the case (e.g., classification and discipline-specific gaps) throughout this chapter we will adopt the term 'athlete selection' when discussing the complexity of this endeavour.

In this chapter, we intend to review the current state of athlete selection and development in Para sport contexts while highlighting directions for future research. To start, we propose a framework for documenting, understanding, and studying the complexity of athlete selection in the context of Para sport. Specifically, we utilize the Institutional Analysis and Design (IAD) framework (Ostrom, 2005; Ostrom et al., 2011). With respect to Para sport, this framework provides a platform to explicitly highlight and categorize the context-specific complexity of athlete selection decisions. Given the nascent state of Para athlete selection literature (Baker et al., 2017), this framework also provides a means to explicitly identify areas for future research. We also hope this framework provides a useful way for practitioners to evaluate decision-making in athlete selection, and, as a result, provide some insight to improve selection processes.

The IAD framework

The IAD framework was created as a tool for understanding situations where decision-makers must make repeated and similar decisions, and it has been used in diverse contexts (Poteete et al., 2010). As highlighted by Hess and Ostrom (2005), IAD is particularly suited to answer questions such as 'How do fallible humans come together, create communities and organizations, and make decisions and rules in order to sustain a resource or achieve a desired outcome?' (pg. 3). Given that decision-makers typically select athletes year-after-year, the IAD framework fits within sporting contexts. Ultimately, however, we believe the IAD framework is valuable because it accurately reflects the different factors and processes involved in decision-making on athlete selection. Research on talent identification and selection can sometimes take a reductionist view of talent selection decisions (i.e., that these decisions are made entirely at an individual level: Lath et al., 2021; Schorer et al., 2017). Alternatively, some research on talent selection accuracy takes a lower fidelity aggregated approach (i.e., aggregating selection decisions across many teams and/or several years of decision-making), effectively removing unique decisions of individuals or groups of individuals from modelling (Farah & Baker, 2021; Koz et al., 2012). The IAD framework emphasizes the interactions between contextual factors and decision-makers, but also the unique inter-individual *dynamics* inherent to athlete selections (as well as the individual characteristics of decision-makers). Thus, our aim is to present the IAD in the context of Para sport athlete selection, and to provide a tool that practitioners can utilize for reflecting on their athlete selection processes.

The IAD framework is not meant to serve as a stand-alone theoretical framework. Instead, it is a meta-theoretical framework (Poteete et al., 2010), wherein other theories and concepts can be embedded. Indeed, to achieve our intended aim and better conceptualize athlete selection elements, we will be incorporating Dehghansai and colleagues' (2020) constraints-led approach to organize these factors within the overarching framework. For the purpose of this chapter, our focus will be on four main sets of variables within the IAD framework (see Figure 5.1): Contextual Variables, the Action Arena, Normative Evaluation Criteria, and Outcomes. For the sake of parsimony, we attempt to present these categories of variables in distinct subsections, but the interactive nature of IAD components necessitates some overlap of topics at times.

Contextual factors

Contextual factors are the variables that are likely to differ from one sport to another, and where there may also be the most notable differences between non-disabled and Para sport settings. Some of these variables may also be the most robustly documented from a research standpoint with respect to development but not selection. Furthermore, *how* these variables influence decision-makers and subsequent athlete selection decisions may be less well understood.

Athlete characteristics[1]

Athlete characteristics include macro- and micro-level elements organized into population size, complexity (i.e., characteristics) and predictability. At a macro level, factors such as the size and availability of the prospective athlete talent pool/population are important because they can influence the amount of information (degrees of freedom) decision-makers have to manage. Naturally, macro athlete characteristics may vary based on population-specific demographics, the rules, and demands of each sport (see *Rules* below), as well as the developmental infrastructure in place for Para sport (see *Infrastructure* below). A recent descriptive study of participants attending a Para sport recruitment event (i.e., a talent search day) found that the majority of participants had some prior experience in sport, and that 65% of participants were male, suggesting such events appeal to some groups more than others (Dehghansai & Baker, 2020). This gap is

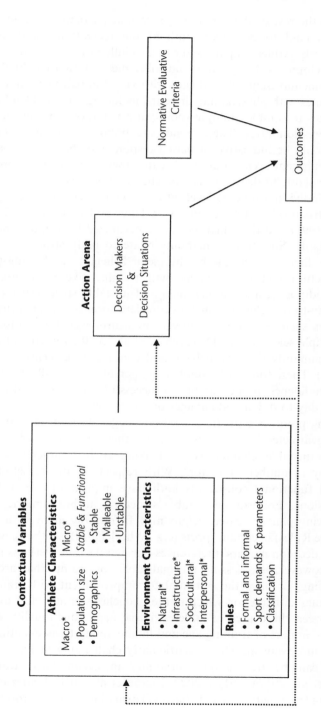

FIGURE 5.1 A constraints-based institutional analysis and design (IAD) framework for athlete selection [* denote variables from Dehghansai et al.'s (2020) constraints-led approach for elite Para sport athlete development]

consistent with the rest of Para sport in general, as participation rates for female athletes tend to be lower, both at the recreational and high-performance levels. Athlete impairment can also influence the selection and subsequent development. Dehghansai and colleagues (2021a, b) highlighted unique developmental trends for athletes with visual impairments in comparison to athletes with physical impairments, including a lower likelihood for these athletes to sample multiple sports, and variations in their developmental progression rates. These trends are important to understand, because they could be indicative of biased responses or barriers to participation in recruitment events, but also because they influence the scope of information available to decision-makers when making selections.

At a more individual (micro) level, athletes' characteristics can be categorized as structural and functional (see Haywood & Getchell, 2009; Newell, 1986, 1991) and these factors can be organized into stable, malleable, and unstable. Structural constraints relate to body structures, and include stable factors such as height, seated height, and wingspan. Malleable structural factors can change with training, like cardiovascular performance, adiposity, and muscle mass and unstable structural factors reflect more day-to-day changes, such as transient soreness or impairment-related changes such as those resulting from neurodegenerative diseases including multiple sclerosis (see Dehghansai et al., 2020). Functional constraints predominantly describe behavioural characteristics (Haywood & Getchell, 2009). These too can be stable (e.g., personality), malleable (e.g., self-efficacy: confidence in one's ability to successfully execute a task), and unstable (e.g., day-to-day mood changes or emotions).

As a starting point, one of the central challenges decision-makers face when selecting athletes is discerning whether they are observing stable, malleable, or unstable characteristics. Parsing these characteristics is complicated by a number of factors. With respect to athlete selection, structural and functional constraints both have implications for athlete selection decisions. For example, stable structural anthropometric constraints like wingspan or seated height may favourably align with task constraints (see Rules) in certain sports (e.g., Wheelchair Basketball), which may influence decision makers' preferences during selection. Perhaps more challenging, however, is assessing the malleable constraints that are the result of training, or have the potential for improvement with training. Thus, it becomes difficult for selectors (i.e., coaches, scouts, etc.) to differentiate between the degree of athletes' impairment functionality while considering the impact of training age and innate ability to assess athletes' potential for improvement. This is particularly challenging in Para sport where there can be tremendous variability in accumulated training (Dehghansai et al., 2017a, 2017b, 2022; Fulton et al., 2010; Lemez et al., 2020), resulting from factors such as (lack of) availability of grassroots and development sport participation opportunities, financial barriers to participation, and athletes' different developmental histories related to their impairment onset (Dehghansai et al., 2020a, 2020b; Patatas et al., 2020). Two athletes with the same level of skill, but dramatically different volumes of accumulated training/experience in the sport may have different levels of potential for future improvement. Athletes' potential trajectories are further impacted by their potential classification, (see Chapter 6 for more on this) which become key components in the selector's assessment framework (i.e., competitiveness of the class, whether the athlete would be at the higher or lower range within the class, etc., Dehghansai et al., 2021c). There are also unstable factors that should be considered, including impairment-related factors which are discussed below.

In scenarios where selection may take place as a one-off discreet event, such as 'come and try days', 'national camps', or national events where coaches and scouts examine athlete performance to decide subsequent developmental opportunities, there is always a risk of mislabelling or attributing an athlete's performance as stable or malleable characteristics, when in fact performance is a manifestation of unstable constraints. For example, an athlete with multiple sclerosis or cerebral palsy may be dealing with impairment-related issues that are impacting their physical or psychological performance on that specific day. Day-to-day challenges with impairments of this nature are common and at times, difficult for persons to control. It may be useful for decision-makers to incorporate mechanisms (e.g., checklists, interviews) so that information about athletes accurately reflects their potential, rather than some unstable (and potentially less relevant) factor (e.g., a day-to-day impairment-related medical complication). Naturally, it would be ideal if evaluations of athletes can be made based on more than one observation.

While impairment-related factors are focal factors informing decisions in Para sport contexts (Dehghansai et al., 2021c; Patatas et al., 2020) and anthropometric and physical characteristics are often the sole focal point in non-disabled contexts (see Johnston et al., 2018), athlete potential and performance are inherently multidimensional (i.e., anthropometric, physiological, psychological, and technical/tactical skill (Johnston & Baker, 2020). As such, decision-makers need to explicitly assess multiple characteristics and weigh this information when evaluating athletes. The micro and macro categorization of population trends are not meant to imply a disparity in the complexity of athlete selection decision-making. On the contrary, micro and macro athlete characteristics simply need to be considered alongside the context-specific *Rules* and *Attributes of Environment* of Para sport, to fully understand the complexity inherent to athlete selection, and to optimize athlete selection strategies. For example, classification criteria (i.e., Rules) may play an exclusionary role in the selection criteria, limiting opportunities for athletes with specific impairments. While, training centre infrastructures may be inaccessible and thus, eliminate chances for certain groups of athletes with specific abilities to access programs and/or events at that venue, reducing opportunities.

Attributes of community

Attributes of the community include a range of variables in the general community in which athletes exist and decision-making takes place. Dehghansai and colleagues (2020) describe four categories of community attributes: natural, infrastructure, sociocultural, and interpersonal. From the perspective of athlete selection, all of these constraints have the potential to facilitate or impede athlete selection decisions. Natural environmental factors, such as geography and physical location, can create barriers (e.g., distance) to participating in sport, attending selection camps/come and try days, or for coaches to travel to see an athlete. For example, Paralympic Search events in Canada typically only occur in large urban centres of some (but not all) provinces. Thus, athletes living in rural regions and/or smaller cities, with limited access to transportation will inevitably have a harder time accessing opportunities to demonstrate their talent to selectors (Dehghansai & Baker, 2020; Radtke & Doll-Tepper, 2014).

Infrastructure

Para sport infrastructures can also vary significantly from one context to another. Even in countries with relatively well-supported infrastructure for high-performance Paralympic sport systems, there are often substantial deficits in grassroots/community development programs. Irrespective of more refined and established sport infrastructures, non-disabled sport still struggles to accurately select talent (i.e., Type I and II errors), and many Paralympic sports do not have these feeder systems to develop talent and filter out athletes with lower potential. Nor is there a way for the developmental system to accommodate the different participation patterns and milestones inherent to athletes in Para sport. This results in a wide variation in skills (and ability) amongst athletes in Para contexts. Moreover, without established structures and systems in place, there are limits imposed on accumulated experience (e.g., sport-specific training, sport sampling), which ultimately impact athletes' development rates. But more importantly, this hinders the quality of many athletes' experiences, for some, removing opportunities altogether. Therefore, we are left with this global issue of low participation rates in Para sport.

Sociocultural

Sociocultural factors describe a broad range of factors distal to the athlete that can influence athletes' selection and development. These include social norms, values, and beliefs, as well as specific policies and laws. Overall, there has been a growing popularization of Paralympic sport with an increase in large international competitions and media recognition (Houlihan & Chapman, 2017). These changes can help promote positive values around Paralympic sport and may impact the popularity of recruitment events (see Dehghansai & Baker, 2020). However, limited funding in the sport system, particularly at developmental levels continues to constrain the system, negatively impacting the sustainability of recruitment events, staffing, and the breadth and diversity of the pool of prospective athletes (Dehghansai et al., 2021c). Indeed, in one study youth participants of an introductory Para sport program lamented that there were limited opportunities for progression, reflecting the gulf that can exist between grassroots and elite high-performance programs (Cavell, 2021).

Interpersonal

The interaction between an individual athlete and their social environment has been well documented. Athletes rely on support and resources from parents, coaches, teammates, and friends to navigate to and around their daily training environments. Indeed, holistic ecological approaches to athlete development suggest alignment between interpersonal supports is essential to successful athlete development programs (Burns et al., 2019). With respect to the selection of athletes, there is some evidence that interpersonal support influences a decision-makers' evaluation of athletes (Dehghansai et al., 2021c). Too much dependence on interpersonal support can be viewed negatively by selectors looking for indicators of independence in athletes. However, too little indication of interpersonal support can also be viewed negatively (because of the logistical and financial resources required to support an athlete). As such, decision-makers may be looking for a 'goldilocks zone' of sorts, where support from family is sufficient to enable the athlete to explore opportunities, but not too much to impede their independence and growth (Dehghansai et al., 2021c; Patatas et al., 2020; Radtke & Doll-Tepper, 2014).

Rules

Rules in some sense act as constraints on the task of decision-making. Rules can be formal (i.e., limits to roster size for international competitions) or informal (e.g., informal agreements, values, and norms), both of which may be sport-specific (see Dehghansai et al., 2020). With respect to

Para sport athlete selection, these rules also encapsulate important sport-specific task constraints (e.g., the parameters and rules of the sport), which can interact with athletes' characteristics to influence selection decisions. For example, seated height and wingspan (stable structural constraints) in Wheelchair Basketball confers a performance advantage. There are also classification-related advantages that may impact selection criteria. For example, Wheelchair Basketball has a 1–4 classification system and a total of 14 points can be on the court at any given time. On the one hand, classification systems have been put in place to create an inclusionary environment where individuals with different abilities can participate in the same environment on a level playing field. However, a selector may be influenced by a need for a specific class when evaluating athletes (see Chapter 6). In addition, a sport may see gaps in a specific class at international events and aim to be strategically selective to develop athletes in that specific class and thereby gain an advantage over their international competition. This practice can create more exclusionary processes within the selection criteria and add another layer of information that selectors utilize in their decision-making process.

Task constraints

There are also task-specific constraints that selectors may consider. These are factors more specific to the execution of skills within a sport (e.g., the ability to navigate around the court and control a racquet to return a ball to the other side of the net). Some confounders that can bias a selector's decision are athletes' training age and their previous experience. As alluded to earlier, in-depth conversations with athletes and attempting to observe athletes on more than one occasion may provide selectors with a deeper understanding of athletes' ability to acquire new skills, their learning progression rate, and demonstrate a baseline to better understand athletes' potential ceiling. Furthermore, there are elements associated with how well an athlete can utilize their abilities to meet sporting demands. For instance, an athlete who just acquired their impairment and recently entered a sport may demonstrate similar skills as to an athlete with a decade's worth of training experience. Limited information on athlete's training age can impact a selector's decision-making on athlete's potential. Thus, the more information readily available and more opportunities to evaluate and assess an athlete can increase the effectiveness of selection.

Action situations

The action arena effectively includes all people making athlete selection decisions. One of the important elements of understanding accurate and inaccurate athlete selection decisions is to know the people involved in decision-making, how much power each person has in decisions rendered (i.e., their roles and positions), their specific decision-making process (e.g., heuristics: Lath et al., 2021), the characteristics that influence their decisions (i.e., preferences, experience, knowledge, biases, and available resources), and the interactions that exist between different people. For example, do selection decisions ultimately rest with one individual, or is decision-making democratized in a team approach? Different sports and organizations may take very different approaches to this decision-making process. Moreover, the cast of actors can be diverse, including a range of people and roles: coaches, assistant coaches, members of integrated support teams, high-performance directors, administrators, athletes in leadership positions, and parents. Furthermore, depending on the specific contexts (geography, infrastructure, level of sport) and macro athlete characteristics, decision-makers may be more involved in recruitment, identification, and/or selection, which may influence the type of decisions they are able to make (Radtke & Doll-Tepper, 2014). If representatives from multiple sports are involved in a recruitment event, like a Paralympian Search (Dehghansai & Baker, 2020), then the action arena may also include competing decision-makers who must negotiate or vie for access to the same athlete. Overall, however, the dynamics of the decision-making process (i.e., number, roles, and characteristics of actors involved) are largely unknown.

From a scientific perspective, little is known about the impact of decision makers' accumulated experience, preferences, and biases with respect to athlete selection in Para sport. As previously mentioned, there are indications that some decision-makers may favour athletes who demonstrate independence from interpersonal supports (though not total independence), have prior sport experience, and family with sport experience (Dehghansai et al., 2021c). More research is needed to better understand if and how other preferences and biases impact selection decisions. Much has been written about the role of cognitive biases in talent selection (see Johnston & Baker, 2020; Till & Baker, 2020), but primarily from a non-disabled sport perspective. For example, what (if any) biases exist for athlete age, certain classifications of impairment, or for athletes with impairments acquired at different stages of their lives (e.g., congenital versus an athlete with impairment acquired in adulthood)? In team sports, it is also not clear whether the characteristics of athletes already on rosters influence evaluations and decision-making strategies about prospective athletes.

Outcomes and normative evaluative criteria

While it is important to understand the contextual variables and decision-making processes related to athlete selection, it is also essential to have a clear articulation of desired and undesired outcomes, and the evaluative criteria used to classify outcomes. Ultimately, most selection decisions related to athlete *potential* result in four outcomes: accurate selection, accurate non-selection, inaccurate selection (type I error; false positive), and inaccurate non-selection (type II error; false negative). The normative evaluative criteria used to understand which of these outcomes has occurred can vary depending on context and decision-makers goals. For decision-makers at grassroots and developmental levels of sport, these normative evaluative criteria may be completely different than those at the elite level. Indeed, evaluative criteria of athlete selections can range from improved skill competency and passion about sport, to personal bests and individual recognitions (e.g., most valuable player awards), overall team performance, improvements in international standings from previous Paralympic cycles, or coveted international championships and Paralympic medals. Nonnormative events (e.g., injury, changes in funding impacting developmental environments/resources) could also influence athletes' developmental trajectories, thus necessitating consideration within the evaluative criteria. If desirable evaluative criteria of athlete selection decisions include *long-term athlete outcomes* (e.g., matriculation to a national team), the time gap between athlete selection decisions and outcomes limit the immediacy of feedback available to decision-makers. The lack of relevant feedback about the accuracy of athlete selection decisions is particularly salient at developmental levels. This is not to suggest long-term goals are inappropriate; rather, relevant short-term processes and evaluative criteria need to be included to create feedback loops. The challenge is identifying short-term evaluative criteria that have valid and reliable predictive utility.

Conclusion

Decision-makers must navigate group dynamics, information and knowledge constraints, and cognitive biases while selecting athletes within a complicated range of environmental and sport-specific constraints. Utilizing this framework, practitioners and researchers can better understand the complexities of athlete selections, and comparisons can be made between more and less successful athlete selection and development programs. In particular, case studies of successful (and less successful) athlete development systems may provide insight into the impact of different decision-making structures. Hypotheses can also be tested utilizing experimental approaches (e.g., modifying rules that govern athlete selection). While we have attempted to summarize current knowledge of athlete selection and development in Para sport contexts, there is a glaring need for more empirical evidence to inform our decisions and enhance the quality of our selection processes.

Practitioner commentary

Based on my experience working in Para sport as both a coach and a practitioner, I found this chapter particularly relevant for those working within Para sport pathways. Para sport can accentuate traditional talent selection issues while also posing additional challenges for a selector's decision-making. The framework provides a good description of the factors that a coach or practitioner should consider when making athlete selection decisions or designing processes within a pathway that will inform athlete selection decisions. A strength of the framework presented is the emphasis on understanding the interaction between factors. For example, there might be an interaction between the following factors:

- an athlete's limited sport-specific training history
- changes to malleable characteristics such as their strength or power
- increased training load because an athlete is selected on to a talent pathway
- classification rules and whether an athlete is at the higher or lower range of a class

In this example, a coach or practitioner may need to consider whether the combination could lead to an athlete becoming ineligible from a classification perspective. Initially, the athlete's strength may fall within the limits for that class/event but this may be due to their limited training history. If the athlete is exposed to an increased training load following selection on to a talent pathway, the athlete's strength may increase and when re-tested their strength may exceed the limits set in the classification rules. A selector will need to consider this possibility when assessing the athlete's talent relative to other athletes. A highly skilled coach or practitioner working in Para sport can identify and consider the opportunities and risks that emerge from the complexity of several interacting factors in a situation like this. Therefore, the framework can help an early-career coach or practitioner identify what factors to consider and how to categorize their observations. However, coaches and practitioners should also remember that no framework can fully capture every possible factor or how they interact. If a coach or practitioner is using the framework to support their decisions, they should also consider what the framework might be missing if using it to think and reflect on a situation.

Selection is only one part of an athlete's development journey. Coaches and practitioners could also consider how this framework might be used to inform performance planning. The framework could help capture the unique combination of factors that relate to an athlete they are working with and identify potential performance gaps and the underlying causes of those gaps. The authors describe how two athletes may have the same level of skill, with dramatically different volumes of accumulated training/experience in the sport. Applying the framework to this situation might allow a coach or practitioner to identify this difference and adapt the individual performance plans for each athlete accordingly. Similarly, a coach or practitioner might be able to use the framework to consider the infrastructure, sociocultural or interpersonal attributes that have led to each athlete's training history/experience. Identifying these attributes may allow for the identification of the most appropriate strategy to bridge an identified performance gap.

Note

1 Originally termed 'Biophysical Conditions', this contextual variable describes the size, complexity and predictability of the athletes being evaluated and selected.

References

Baker, J., Lemez, S., Van Neutegem, A., & Wattie, N. (2017). Talent selection and development in parasport. In J. Baker, S. Cobley, J. Schorer & N. Wattie (Eds.), *The Routledge handbook of talent identification and development in sport* (pp. 432–442). London: Routledge.

Baker, J., & Wattie, N. (2018). Innate talent in sport: Separating myth from reality. *Current Issues in Sport Science*, 3(6), 1–9.

Baker, J., Wattie, N., & Schorer, J. (2019). A proposed conceptualization of talent in sport: The first step in a long and winding road. *Psychology of Sport Exercise*, 43(7), 27–33.

Baker, J., Wilson, S., Johnston, K., Dehghansai, N., Koenigsberg, A., De Vegt, S., & Wattie, N. (2020). Talent research in sport 1990–2018: A scoping review. *Frontiers in Psychology*, 11, 607710.

Burns, L., Weissensteiner, J. R., & Cohen, M. (2019). Supportive interpersonal relationships: A key component to high-performance sport. *British Journal of Sports Medicine*, 53(22), 1386–1389.

Cavell, M. (2021). Experiences in a multi-sport Parasport program: The female adolescent perspective. Master's thesis, OntarioTech University, https://ir.library.dc-uoit.ca/handle/10155/1201

Collins, D., McNamara, A., & Cruickshank, A. (2019). Research and practice in talent identification and development – Some thoughts on the state of play. *Journal of Applied Sport Psychology*, 31(3), 340–351.

Dehghansai, N., & Baker, J. (2020). Searching for Paralympians: Characteristics of participants attending "Search" events. *Adapted Physical Activity Quarterly*, 37(1), 129–138.

Dehghansai, N., Allan, V., Pinder, R., & Baker, J. (2021a). The impact of athletes' impairment type on their developmental trajectories. *Adapted Physical Activity Quarterly*, 39(1), 129–138.

Dehghansai, N., Pinder, R. A., & Baker, J. (2022). Pathways in Paralympic sport: An in-depth analysis of athletes' developmental trajectories and training histories. *Adapted Physical Activity Quarterly, 39*(1), 37–85.

Dehghansai, N., Pinder, R. A., & Baker, J. (2021c). "Looking for a golden needle in the haystack": Perspectives on talent identification and development in Paralympic sport. *Frontiers in Sports & Active Living, 3,* 635977.

Dehghansai, N., Lemez, S., Wattie, N., & Baker, J. (2017a). A systematic review of influences on para-athlete development. *Adapted Physical Activity Quarterly, 34*(1), 72–90.

Dehghansai, N., Lemez, S., Wattie, N., & Baker, J. (2017b). Training and development of Canadian wheelchair basketball players. *European Journal of Sport Science, 17*(5), 511–518.

Dehghansai, N., Lemez, S., Wattie, N., Pinder, R. A., & Baker, J. (2020a). Understanding the development of elite parasport athletes using a constraint-led approach: Considerations for coaches and practitioners. *Frontiers in Psychology, 11,* 502981.

Dehghansai, N., Spedale, D., Wilson, M. J., & Baker, J. (2020b). Comparing Developmental Trajectories of Elite Able-Bodied and Wheelchair Basketball Players. *Adapted Physical Activity Quarterly, 37*(3), 338–348.

Farah, L., & Baker, J. (2021). Accuracy from the slot: Evaluating draft selections in the National Hockey League. *Scandinavian Journal of Medicine & Science in Sports, 31,* 564–572.

Fulton, S. K., Pyne, D. B., Hopkins, W. G., & Burkett, B. (2010). Training characteristics of Paralympic swimmers. *Journal of Strength and Conditioning Research, 24*(2), 471–478.

Gerrard, B. (2017). The role of analytics in assessing playing talent. In J. Baker, S. Cobley, J. Schorer & N. Wattie (Eds.), *The Routledge handbook of talent identification and development in sport* (pp. 423–431). London: Routledge.

Haywood, K. M., & Getchell, N. (2009). *Life span motor development* (5th ed.). Champaign: Human Kinetics.

Hess, C., & Ostrom, E. (2005). A framework for analyzing the knowledge commons: A chapter from understanding knowledge as a commons: From theory to practice. *Libraries' and Librarians' Publications, 21,* 1–54.

Houlihan, B., & Chapman, P. (2017). Talent identification and development in elite youth disability sport. *Sport in Society, 20*(1), 107–125.

Howe, M. J. A., Davidson, J. W., & Sloboda, J. A. (1998). Innate talents: Reality or myth? *Behavior & Brain Science, 21*(3), 399–442.

Johnston, K., & Baker, J. (2020). Waste reduction strategies: Factors affecting talent wastage and the efficacy of talent selection in sport. *Frontiers in Psychology, 10,* 2925.

Johnston, K., Wattie, N., Schorer, J., & Baker, J. (2018). Talent identification in sport: A systematic review. *Sports Medicine, 48*(1), 97–109.

Koz, D., Fraser-Thomas, J., & Baker, J. (2012). Accuracy of professional sports drafts in predicting career potential. *Scandinavian Journal of Medicine & Science in Sports, 22*(4), 64–69.

Lath, F., Hartigh, R., Wattie, N., & Schorer, J. (2021). Talent selection: Making decisions and prognoses about athletes. In J. Baker, S. Cobley, & J. Schorer (Eds.), *Talent identification and development in sport: International perspectives* (2nd ed., pp. 50–65). Routledge.

Lemez, S., Wattie, N., Dehghansai, N., & Baker, J. (2020). Developmental pathways of Para athletes: Examining the sporting backgrounds of elite Canadian wheelchair basketball players. *Current Issues in Sport Science, 5,* 002.

Newell, K. (1986). Constraints on the development of coordination. In M. G. Wade, & H. T. A. Whiting (Eds.), *Motor development in children: Aspects of coordination and control* (pp. 341–360). Dordrecht: Martinus Nijhoff.

Newell, K. M. (1991). Motor skill acquisition. *Annual Review of Psychology, 42,* 213–217.

Ostrom, E. (2005). *Understanding institutional diversity.* Princeton: Princeton University Press.

Ostrom, E., Gardner, R., & Walker, J. (2011). *Rules, games, & common-pool resources.* Michigan: The University of Michigan Press.

Patatas, J. M., De Bosscher, V., Derom, I., & Winckler, C. (2020). Stakeholders' perceptions of athletic career pathways in Paralympic sport: From participant to excellence. *Sport Science, 25*(2), 299–320.

Poteete, A. R., Janssen, M. A., & Ostrom, E. (2010). *Working together: Collective action, the commons, and multiple methods in practice.* Princeton: Princeton University Press.

Radtke, S., & Doll-Tepper, G. (2014). *A cross-cultural comparison of talent identification and development in Paralympic sports.* Cologne: Sportverlag.

Schorer, J., Rienhoff, R., Fischer, L., & Baker, J. (2017). Long-term prognostic validity of talent selections: Comparing national and regional coaches, laypersons and novices. *Frontiers, 8,* 1146.

Till, K., & Baker, J. (2020). Challenges and [possible] solutions to optimizing talent identification and development in sport. *Frontiers in Psychology, 11,* 664.

6

THE ROLE OF CLASSIFICATION IN TALENT IDENTIFICATION AND DEVELOPMENT IN PARA SPORTS

Daniel Fortin-Guichard, Eline Blaauw, Ralf van der Rijst, Sean Tweedy, and David Mann
Practitioner Commentary: Michael Woods

Talent identification in Para sports is directionless without classification. Take for instance a Wheelchair Track athlete who can race 100 m in 18.5 sec. That athlete would have won a medal at the Tokyo 2020 Paralympic Games in the 100 m final of the T33 class, a class for athletes with moderate to severe impairment of both legs and at least one arm. The athlete would be an outstanding prospect. However, that same athlete would not have even met the minimum entry standard for the Tokyo Games if classified in the T34 class designed for those with largely lower-limb impairment. That athlete might never be competitive internationally, or even nationally, even with extensive support. Accordingly, it is not possible to know how talented a Para athlete is in a particular sport – let alone their potential for *future* success – without knowledge of that Para sport's classification system and how an athlete's impairment would be evaluated under that system.

Classification helps to create fairer competition in all sports. Athletes are typically classified so that they compete against others based on characteristics known to impact performance such as sex or weight (e.g., in combat sports). In Para sport, classification places athletes into classes based on the extent to which their particular impairment profile – type, severity, and distribution – will adversely affect performance in their chosen sport. The overarching aim of Para sport classification is to maximise the likelihood that the outcome of competition depends on talent, training, and motivation, rather than on the basis of who has the least impairment (Tweedy & Vanlandewijck, 2011). This aim is essential, but in practice, can be very challenging to achieve. And the failure to achieve this aim can have

DOI: 10.4324/9781003184430-6

significant implications for the way that high-performance programs identify talent (Spathis et al., 2015).

There are typically four key steps in the process of classification for Para athletes. The first step requires the athlete to supply medical documentation which confirms that they have a health condition that could potentially cause one or more of the ten impairment types that would make an athlete eligible to compete in Paralympic sport (each is either a physical, visual, or intellectual impairment; see Tweedy et al., 2016). When the athlete presents for classification, a classification panel is responsible for conducting the remaining three steps. First, the panel must confirm that the athlete has an eligible impairment. For example, some types of spina bifida (e.g., occulta) can be completely asymptomatic, and in such a case the athlete would not be eligible. However, if the athlete has muscle power impairment that is consistent with their diagnosis, then the panel undertakes the next step which is to determine whether the severity of their impairment meets the *minimum impairment criteria* (MIC) for their chosen sport. Each Para sport develops its own MIC, which is set with the aim of ensuring that athletes qualify only if they have an impairment that adversely affects their performance in that sport. Finally, athletes who meet the MIC are allocated a *sport class* so that they compete against others who share characteristics known to impact performance similarly (International Paralympic Committee, 2007; 2015). In other words, each Para sports class should comprise athletes who have impairments that cause a comparable amount of difficulty in that sport.

The way that classification systems have been designed has changed markedly over the past 20 years. Originally, athletes were classified based on their medical diagnosis. For instance, within a given sport, there may have been a class for athletes with a spinal cord injury, a class for lower limb amputations, and another class for athletes with short stature. A problem with this method is that it did not necessarily consider the severity of each athlete's impairment on their sport performance (Tweedy & Vanlandewijck, 2011). For instance, the activity limitations for an athlete with a high-level spinal cord injury would be much more severe than those for an athlete with a lower-level injury. Moreover, it is possible that two athletes even with the same level of injury could have different activity limitations. Because of these shortcomings, the International Paralympic Committee (IPC) mandated, in establishing the *Athlete Classification Code* (International Paralympic Committee, 2007; 2015), a move towards *evidence-based classification* in Para sport. Evidence-based classification requires a classification system to be based on empirical evidence which uncovers the relationship between impairment and sport performance. As a result, under evidence-based classification, it is possible that athletes with very different health conditions could compete against each other *if* the impact of their impairment on sport performance is comparable. Vitally, the impact of impairment on performance is likely to differ according to the demands of the sport in question. For instance, an upper limb impairment may have a profound effect on an athlete's swimming ability, but only limited effect on their ability to ski or play football. Therefore, an evidence-based system of classification is also necessarily sport specific. Not only will the classes be different across sports, so too will the MIC, meaning that an athlete with impairment might qualify to compete in some sports, but not in others (Tweedy & Vanlandewijck, 2011; Vanlandewijck & Thompson, 2010).

Although the move towards evidence-based classification is necessary, weaknesses still remain. The research required to underpin evidence-based classification requires time and resources, meaning that some sports continue to use an outdated system that lacks evidence. Other sports have made initial changes and would benefit from further refinements to their classification system (Mann et al., 2021). Collectively, there is a considerable chance that those sports continue to rely on a system whereby the impact of impairment on performance is not well understood and so athletes with a lower level of impairment may have a competitive advantage over others in their class.

Even when the impairment-performance relationship and ideal sport class structure is known for a given sport, other practical limitations mean that some athletes might retain an advantage within an evidence-based system. For instance, an 'ideal' class structure might require more classes than is practically possible, either because there would not be enough athletes to generate sufficient competition within those classes, and/or if there is a limitation in the number of medal events that a sport can offer (e.g., only a limited number of medals can be awarded at any one Paralympic Games). In those cases, classes may need to be combined, or athletes may need to compete 'up' in a class designed for others with less impairment if their own class is not offered. These weaknesses in existing classification systems can have significant consequences for the way that sport organisations identify talent in Para sports, a point we return to shortly.

What happens during classification?

In order to compete at an international competition in Para sport, athletes need to be evaluated by internationally recognized classifiers (Vanlandewijck & Thompson, 2010). Classification procedures vary depending on the type of impairment. In a sport designed for athletes with a physical impairment, classification is mainly determined by the level of coordination, range of motion and/or muscle power of the affected limb(s), as well as the level of function during sport participation (International Paralympic Committee, 2020). For athletes with vision impairment, classification is based on the severity of an athlete's vision loss. Their impairment can be caused by damage to the eye structure, optic nerves, optical pathways, or visual cortex. Classification in vision impairment is not yet sport-specific, with classification determined by measuring an athlete's visual acuity and/or their visual field (with rifle shooting being the first exception; Allen et al., 2016; 2018; 2019; Latham et al., 2021; Myint et al., 2016; World Shooting Para Sport, 2019 and now judo; Krabben, Mashkovskiy, et al. 2021; Krabben, Ravensbergen, et al., 2021). For athletes with intellectual impairment, classification is based on how everyday life activities are impacted by conceptual, social, and practical skills, and how these restrictions in intellectual functioning and adaptive behaviours impact sport performance. Classification of an athlete with intellectual impairment is based on results of tests of sport cognition (Van Biesen et al., 2021).

The relationship between classification and talent identification

Talent identification is the process of recognizing individuals with the potential to excel in a sport in the future (Baker et al., 2013; Vaeyens et al., 2008). In non-disabled sports, talent identification is performed largely by determining the key components of performance in a certain sport (e.g., speed, strength, technical abilities) and then searching for individuals with those abilities or those who may have the potential to develop them in the future. Sports may further tailor their search criteria depending on their own classification systems (e.g., on the basis of an individual's age and gender). For instance, in a sport where vertical jump height is important, gender-specific normative data for vertical jump may be vital. A 40 cm jump height would be highly impressive for an adult female, but not at all for a male (Patterson & Peterson, 2004). Indeed, a woman in the 90th percentile would not make it to the 10th percentile among men. But in general, sports would be interested in recruiting any individual who has better capabilities than the rest of the population.

In Para sport however, only a limited sub-set of the wider population will qualify to compete and therefore an evaluation of impairment is typically a vital step – and sometimes the first step – in the talent identification process (Diaper, 2015; Spathis et al., 2015). The existence of MIC in Para sports means that only some individuals will ever qualify to compete in the sport. Accordingly, sport organizations such as National sport or Paralympic federations who seek to identify future Paralympians may be interested only in athletes who will qualify to compete internationally in the Para sport. While this may not be a concern for talent search programs that are not interested in performance at international or even national competitions (e.g., for those seeking to enhance participation at a community level), it is a vital consideration for programs that will be evaluated on (inter)national performance. Those programs might receive no direct benefit from identifying and supporting athletes who cannot compete in the sports they govern (see Chapter 4 for impact of this on recruitment and identification and Chapter 14 for sociocultural influences).

Caution is warranted when performing this first evaluation of an athlete's impairment. Those running Para sport talent identification programs have an important role to play in ensuring that prospective athletes are educated so that they understand that meeting the MIC is a requirement of participating in Para sport and that the MIC are largely sport-specific, so the athlete might be eligible for one sport and ineligible for another (e.g., through-hand amputation is eligible for swimming but not for athletics). Vitally, the failure to meet the MIC does not mean that the athlete does not have an impairment. Rather it means that they do not have an impairment which fits into the competition structure for that Para sport. Good talent ID programs should make provision for guiding opportunities for athletes who are not eligible for sports opportunities.

It is noteworthy that the interest in talent identification programs may extend to individuals who *do not yet* meet the MIC but might in the future if/when their impairment progresses. Indeed, although some health conditions lead to impairments that are stable and not training responsive (e.g., short stature, amputation), other types of impairments are either progressive (e.g., multiple sclerosis and some genetic eye disorders) or training responsive (e.g., cerebral palsy), inviting sport organizations to plan ahead and target those athletes who may end up eligible. There are however risks associated with this approach. First, an individual's impairment might not progress at the rate expected and so they might not meet the MIC until much later in their life (if at all). Second, athletes in this situation anecdotally talk sometimes about the irony and mental burden of essentially waiting for their impairment to become worse so they can qualify to compete. Finally, training responsiveness means that the functional ability of some untrained individuals with physical impairment can improve as a result of training. This means that an individual who just fails to meet the MIC might move even further from it if their functional ability improves with training. Clearly, there are risks associated with identifying athletes whose impairment sits close to the MIC.

While some sport federations are interested only in those athletes who meet the MIC for a sport, this is not always the case. Nations sometimes implement classification rules that are more inclusive than those used internationally to encourage more individuals with an impairment to participate in local competitions. As noted, it might be that the national federation wants to provide competition opportunities for individuals whose impairment may progress to meet the MIC sometime in the future

(Tweedy & Vanlandewijck, 2011). However, a national federation might also want to encourage those with less impairment to participate, either to create enough competition for those who do qualify to compete internationally, or more simply to provide opportunities for more individuals with impairment to participate in sport for their own wider health and psychosocial benefits. Therefore, national classification systems sometimes introduce additional classes to help include those potential athletes and to generate more competition (Powis & MacBeth, 2020). These athletes would be missed by coaches and scouts if only the international rules were to be followed during talent identification.

When a prospective athlete does meet the MIC to take part in a Para sport, then their talent still needs to be evaluated *relative to* their level of impairment. As the example presented in the opening of this chapter illustrates, a certain level of performance in wheelchair racing over a distance of 100 m may be very promising for an athlete with severe physical activity limitation, but less so for an athlete with less severe limitation. This means that those responsible for talent identification programs must be very familiar with the classification system of the sport(s) for which they are seeking talent. This process can provide an indication of the athlete's likely sport class so that a judgement can be made of a prospective athlete's talent, though only the actual classification process will give the final answer. Sport organizations could for instance work with National Classifiers to provide a more accurate assessment of a potential athlete's likely sport class.

Given the move towards sport-specific classification, talent identification can be increasingly complex for multi-sport programs that search for individuals on behalf of a group of different sports. Multi-sport identification programs such as the highly successful 'Talentdagen' run by the Netherlands Olympic and Paralympic Committee (NOC*NSF) attract and test individuals with impairment with an aim to match those with athletic potential to a sport program that suits their interests and capabilities. Programs such as these must evaluate each individual's impairment relative to the classification system for each sport of interest. This allows a determination of which sports the individual might qualify to compete in, and for those for which they would qualify, to evaluate the individual's potential relative to their impairment. Accordingly, some sport organizations such as NOC*NSF consider an evaluation of impairment to be the *first step* required in talent identification in multi-sport Para sport programs.

Sometimes, classification requirements also lead sports to search for athletes with a particular type and/or level of impairment. This is particularly the case in those Para team sports such as Wheelchair Basketball and VI cricket in which teams must consist of athletes across a range of sport classes. For instance, in Wheelchair Rugby, all players' impairments are classified on a point system from 0.5 to 3.5 (from most to least impaired). Only four players are allowed on court at any one time, and the sum of the points for all four players must be 8 points or less (International Wheelchair Rugby Federation, 2021). So, a team may have two extremely good '3.5- points' players, but would only be able to have them on court at the same time as two 0.5 players. Accordingly, the team may prioritize identifying individuals with a class of 0.5 to ensure they can field their talented 3.5-points players. In essence, that team would be searching for players with specific levels of impairment because of the constraints placed on them by classification.

It is also possible that individuals with less impairment may be identified to play specific roles within a team. For example, in visual impairment cricket, athletes with less impairment may be identified not necessarily because they are more skilled, but rather because their visual ability is more suitable for fielding on the boundary of the ground, far from the action, because they can see the ball from further distances than others can (Powis & MacBeth, 2020).

Exploiting weaknesses in a classification system

Some use talent identification to gain a competitive advantage by exploiting weaknesses in existing classification systems. As noted, some sports continue to use an outdated classification system that might result in considerable differences in the activity limitations of athletes within classes. For instance, VI judo for many years used only one sport class, yet there is considerable evidence to show that those athletes who are completely blind are at a disadvantage when competing against athletes with some remaining vision (Krabben et al., 2018; 2021) and with subsequently less likely to win medals at international competitions (Kons et al., 2019; 2021). Accordingly, national federations may seek to identify athletes with less impairment given that it is known that they will have an advantage during competition. Some may even consider it to be illogical to recruit blind athletes unless their ability was so outstanding that it would compensate for their competitive disadvantage.

Targeting athletes close to cut-offs

Even when an evidence-based system of classification is implemented, classification cannot entirely eliminate the impact of impairment on the outcome of competition. In those cases, incentive remains for federations to identify athletes with less impairment, because those athletes may have a competitive advantage against others with more impairment within their class. Classification requires choices to be made that strike a balance between creating as many classes as is necessary to maximise fairness, while at the same time not creating so many classes that it decreases the value of winning a medal when too many medals are awarded. Therefore, even within an evidence-based system, each sport class can cover a range of impairment levels that might not entirely have an equitable impact on sport performance. When differences remain within classes regarding athletes' activity limitations, federations have an incentive to favor the identification of those athletes with a beneficial level of impairment when competing in that class. This generally results in sport federations targeting athletes who just meet the MIC for that sport or whose impairment is just within the cut-off for a certain class.

Targeting athletes with low and high-support needs

Even without the impact of classification, an athlete's level of impairment might still impact the likelihood that they are identified and recruited into a high-performance Para sport program. Athletes with high-support needs (e.g., those with a motor-complete cervical level spinal cord injury or those completely blind) by nature require more human and/or financial resources to remain active within a high-performance program. For instance, they might require their own personal support staff, accessible accommodation and training facilities, and individualized training and travel arrangements (Dutia & Tweedy, 2021). Given that national and regional sport federations have limitations on the resources available to them, there remains an incentive for those federations to identify athletes with less impairment because it will be cheaper and easier to support those athletes. Effectively, a federation with limited resources can support more athletes, and potentially increase their chance of winning medals, by identifying those with less impairment. This in itself can represent a threat to the legitimacy of the Para sport movement because it would ultimately result in competition largely for those with less impairment and would deny opportunities to those with high-support needs for whom the Paralympic movement was largely originally designed.

Sport federations may need to be incentivized to recruit athletes with high-support needs. For instance, teams could be required to include a particular proportion of athletes classified as having high-support needs. The IPC's Strategic Plan (International Paralympic Committee, 2019) explicitly seeks to safeguard competition for athletes with high-support needs when forced to make choices about which sport classes to include in the Paralympic program (e.g., VI football is offered in the Paralympic program only for B1 athletes who are essentially blind and not for those with some remaining vision). Even without any explicit requirements or quotas, incentives remain for the astute federation. For instance, talent identification can be less complex for athletes with high-support needs because the targeted population is smaller. Moreover, a committed athlete with high-support needs who has available the necessary personal support and financial resources to train may be more likely to be successful than an athlete with less impairment given that there are often fewer competitors within those classes. Finally, athletes with high-support needs are often among the most inspiring and admired Para sport athletes. Sport federations can benefit and grow with high-support needs athletes as significant role models on their team (Pérez-Torralba et al., 2019).

Why might classification impact talent development?

If classification impacts talent identification, then naturally it will also influence talent *development* in Para sports. Once an athlete has been identified as being 'talented' or as a 'Paralympic potential' (e.g., NOC*NSF, 2021), then sport organizations often seek to develop that talent through the provision of structured support and/or learning environments to help the athlete to realize their potential in the sport (Baker et al., 2013; Vaeyens et al., 2008). Therefore, athletes who are identified as talented will receive access to resources and support that would not otherwise have been available to them if not identified. The impact of these benefits can be substantial given the specific barriers to talent development in Para sports (e.g., difficulties in accessing training facilities, minimal competition opportunities; Baker et al., 2017; Mann et al., 2017). Identified athletes continue to benefit through access to resources, while de-identified athletes do not and may develop their talent at a much slower rate, or may drop out of sport entirely.

A parallel can be drawn between classification and junior age competitions in the way that each can impact talent development in sport. Age grouping (e.g., Under-9s, 10 s, 11 s) is used to structure junior sports so that children play against others of a similar age and therefore presumably skill and maturation level. However, the use of hard cut-off dates for inclusion in an under-age competition (usually January 1st or September 1st) means that differences still exist in the ages of those children playing with and against each other. These differences are understood to result in relative age effects (Barnsley et al. 1985; Cobley et al., 2009; Grondin et al., 1984; Musch & Grondin, 2001), where children born just after the cut-off date are more likely to succeed than those born later in the selection year. Relatively older children are more likely to be judged as being better at the sport (both by their own judgments and those of others such as coaches and scouts) and as a result, may invest in their own development, and/or may be identified as being talented and given access to resources and coaching that others do not. Accordingly, those born soon after the cut-off date are more likely to be over-represented in junior representative teams, but also in senior teams long after age cut-offs are no longer employed. Relatively younger children do not receive the same benefits and are increasingly more likely to drop out of the sport altogether (Helsen et al., 1998).

Classification may impact talent development in a manner that is similar to the relative age effect. Those Para athletes who within their class are less impaired than others may be identified as talented and/or likely to be selected into a talent pathway if others perceive that they will have a competitive advantage or are easier to support. Those athletes may then enjoy better access to training opportunities, including better coaching, equipment and financial support (e.g., for traveling to competition, salary for coaches). Those athletes can therefore focus on training and maximize their chance of fulfilling their athletic potential. On the other hand, deselected athletes inevitably miss out on those crucial opportunities and instead must find their own resources. Spending time searching for financial support and quality coaches rather than training may impact their learning process, or could more simply lead to drop-out from sports entirely. Accordingly, athletes disadvantaged by their classification status may be even further disadvantaged if they have reduced learning opportunities.

While classification appears to impact talent development, the converse is also true: talent development can impact the ability to develop evidence-based classification systems. Evidence-based classification is developed largely through studying the relationship between impairment and performance in Paralympic athletes (Mann & Ravensbergen, 2018; Tweedy & Vanlandewijck, 2011; Van Biesen et al., 2021). For instance, when trying to establish an appropriate class structure for Para Swimming for athletes with physical impairment, evidence-based classification should seek to recruit well-trained international Para swimmers to quantify their physical impairment, and to measure their functional ability on tests that represent determinants of performance in swimming (e.g., the ability to kick and/or rotate at the shoulder). And ideally, athletes should be recruited in a way that ensures there is a valid representative sample of the different levels of severity of impairment that exist in the wider population (e.g., all different levels of spinal cord injury). However, a representative sample of athletes who are well trained might not always exist. In particular, weaknesses in the *existing* classification system might result in an under-representation of athletes whose impairment is disadvantageous under that system. Indeed, if there is a particular level of impairment that is (*perceived to be*) disadvantageous within an existing class, then there is likely to be an under-representation or even absence of athletes who have that level of impairment. And even if there are athletes who are competing with that level of impairment, they may be less well-trained because they have poorer access to resources and support. Accordingly, it is difficult in evidence-based classification research to determine whether athletes with that level of impairment do indeed perform poorer as a result of a greater activity limitation than others in their class (in which case they should ideally be allocated to a different class or their own class), or rather whether they do not have a disadvantage and might perform as well as the other athletes in the class given appropriate access to resources to develop their talent. Accordingly, biases in talent development under an existing classification system hinder our ability to fully understand the relationship between impairment and performance because it results in an under-representation of athletes with that type of impairment and leaves gaps in the continuum of impairment (Fortin-Guichard et al., 2022; Krabben, Ravensbergen et al., 2021; Stalin et al., 2021).

Factors that might impact talent development that classification does not (currently) account for

Another important issue to consider in talent development is the degree to which an athlete's impairment can impact their ability to acquire skill in a sport in a way that classification cannot account for. Classification seeks to establish the impact of impairment on performance *during competition only* (Tweedy & Vanlandewijck, 2011) and does not seek to account for any impact on the ability to acquire skill outside of competition. Yet, the degree of an athlete's impairment can differentially impact their ability to acquire skill as a result of training (Ravensbergen et al., 2016). For instance, it can be challenging for athletes with more severe impairment to simply attend training. While an athlete with vision impairment with some remaining vision may still be able to take public transport or even in some countries to drive to a training venue, an athlete who is blind may be less capable and could require a guide to assist them. Similarly, an athlete with a more severe physical impairment may require special transportation and may not be able to use public transport, particularly if the transport is not accessible (e.g., wheelchair-accessible platforms). In essence, from a talent development perspective, the ability to develop an athlete's talent might be constrained by the severity of their impairment and have a greater impact on athletes with more severe impairment.

Even during training, an athlete's ability to acquire skills might be further impacted by their level of impairment. Again, fully blind athletes may require a guide (e.g., in Para Athletics, Para Skiing or Para Triathlon) or a 'tapper' to provide physical feedback about when to turn when swimming, whereas an athlete with remaining vision might not. Despite these relative disadvantages for those with more severe impairments, they are generally *not* accounted for during classification. The general rationale appears to be that it is already overly complex to design a classification system on the basis of the relationship between impairment and performance *during* competition. It would most likely add an unrealistic layer of complexity to classification systems if they tried to account for any additional impact of the impairment *outside* of competition. From a talent development perspective, again, it may be more challenging for those with more impairment to reach their true potential.

Congenital versus acquired impairment

The age at which an athlete has acquired their impairment is another factor that can impact talent development but is not currently addressed during classification. This is particularly relevant for athletes with vision impairment. It remains possible that two hypothetical athletes with the same level of vision impairment could have very different levels of performance depending on when they acquired that impairment (Mann & Ravensbergen, 2018; Ravensbergen et al., 2016; Tweedy et al., 2016). In some cases, it could be advantageous to have a congenital impairment (i.e., one present since birth). For instance, it could be that a shooter born without vision is more adjusted to their impairment than another athlete who recently lost their vision, and in particular they may be better able to exploit auditory information that is used to guide the gun barrel in VI shooting. On the other hand, a swimmer who acquired a vision impairment later in life may have an advantage over an opponent born blind if they were able to learn to perform both basic motor skills and a complex swimming action with the benefit of vision prior to acquiring their impairment. Again, classification does not at present account for the age at which an impairment is acquired, and it is unclear if it would ever be possible to consider it. Because classification should only account for the impact of impairment on performance during competition, then one interpretation is that classification cannot and should not account for the ability to acquire skill. Conversely, if it were to be shown that the age at which an impairment is acquired impacts an athlete's fundamental ability to acquire skill, then an argument could be made that classification should account for that impairment. To date, there has been insufficient evidence to demonstrate that a congenital impairment differentially impacts skill performance. Again, this could be because congenital impairments are indeed rare, or it could be because they do have a greater impairment in their ability to acquire skill. Further evidence is needed to test the impact of congenital impairments and to subsequently decide whether this is a factor that should be accounted for during classification and so are under-represented at international competitions.

Conclusion

Effective talent identification is simply not possible in Para sports without knowledge about that sport's classification system. Sport federations are in most cases only likely to want to identify athletes who meet a sport's MIC, though the recruitment of those who do not meet the criteria can increase the overall level of competition nationally and provide opportunities for those whose impairment might progress. For those who do meet the criteria, an athlete's potential should be evaluated relative to their likely sport class. Sports do sometimes seek to identify athletes from specific sport classes if they are needed (e.g., for the optimal composition of team sports), and those requirements will change if a classification system changes. If there are weaknesses in a classification system, some sport federations may seek to take advantage by specifically recruiting athletes who they perceive to have a competitive advantage within their sport class such as those who just meet the MIC. This highlights the need for strong evidence-based classification systems to minimize any relationship between impairment and performance within a class and therefore to mitigate any incentives for federations to search for athletes with the least impairment within a class.

Practitioner commentary

A talented athlete in Para sport is not just about having desirable physical, technical, and tactical capabilities, it is very much influenced by where an athlete falls within the sport's classification system. In most cases, the talent pool is very small, hundreds of potential athletes, maybe less. While this means there are fewer athletes to choose from compared to many thousands in non-disabled sports, this also means Para programs can have visibility on most, if not all, athletes in the pipeline. This pipeline starts with classification, but classification has a role beyond the entry point.

Accurate and timely classification places an athlete's performance in context. First, it enables comparison of performance and capabilities with peers at the same developmental stage, with the whole athlete cohort and with the various benchmarks and thresholds built into the development pathway. Second and more importantly, it provides qualification and selection standards in high-performance contexts to ultimately answer the question, does this athlete have medal potential?

The key here is to obtain an accurate classification at the earliest stage possible.

For me, classification serves multiple purposes – the gateway into disability sport, the structure for fair and meaningful competition and the framework for identification of talent to fuel the high-performance pipeline. There can be tension between these objectives and balancing priorities can present a challenge. Less advanced Para sport programs often fail to realize the vital connection between classification and athlete development and ultimately podium success at a Paralympic Games. In domestic classification programs, there is often a focus solely on classification service delivery – getting athletes classified so they can participate in competition.

However, domestic classification systems must also be aligned to the athlete's stage of development, progression in the competitive pathway and as a means to prepare talented athletes for international classification. When this system is combined with a strong framework of performance standards required for high performance it enables talented athletes to be identified.

Talent identification in Para sport needs to be viewed as an ecosystem, not an isolated program. Classification forms the spine of that eco-system interconnected with development stages, pathway programs, and high-performance monitoring and support activities. This includes:

- Strong domestic (national) classification service delivery aligned to international rules and standards
- Clear performance standards for each classification aligned to high-performance benchmarks.
- Regular monitoring of individual athlete classification outcomes and performances
- Regular monitoring of the athlete cohort to identify gaps and opportunities related to medal opportunities at the Paralympic Games and other benchmark competitions.
- Strong system of athlete preparation and support through international classification aligned to the cycle of international benchmark competition.

When delivered successfully, this eco-system leads to significant benefits for Para sport programs. It allows athletes to progress through the pathway with confidence and clarity while providing high-performance programs a high degree of confidence in an athlete's potential. This enables efficient and effective allocation of support including investments and service delivery to enhance an athlete's prospects. This leads to higher conversion rates from pre-elite programs into high-performance programs and ultimately podium results. Equally, it can give rise to rapid progression of talented athletes. Once established you can let the ecosystem do its job. But this requires adequate and ongoing resourcing. It requires strong policies, procedures, protocols, and experienced personnel. Those Para sport programs that can effectively connect classification into their talent identification strategy will find itself with a competitive advantage over their rivals on the world stage.

References

Allen, P., Latham K., Mann D. L., Ravensbergen R. H., & Myint, J. (2016). The level of vision necessary for competitive performance in rifle shooting: Setting the standards for Paralympic shooting with vision impairment. *Frontiers in Psychology*, 7, 1731.

Allen, P., Latham, K., Ravensbergen, R. H., Myint, J., & Mann, D. L. (2019). Rifle shooting for athletes with vision impairment: Does one class fit all? *Frontiers in Psychology, 10*, 1727.

Allen, P., Ravensbergen, R. H., Latham, K., Rose, A., Myint, J., & Mann, D. L. (2018). Contrast sensitivity is a significant predictor of performance in rifle shooting for athletes with vision impairment. *Frontiers in Psychology, 9*, 950.

Baker, J., Cobley, S., & Schorer, J. (2013). *Talent identification and development in sport: International perspectives.* Routledge: Abingdon, UK.

Baker, J., Lemez, S., Van Neutegem, A., & Wattie, N. (2017). Talent development in parasport. In Baker, J., Cobley, S., Schorer, J., & Wattie, N. (Eds.), *Routledge handbook of talent identification and development in sport* (pp. 432–442). Routledge.

Barnsley R. H., Thompson A. H., & Barnsley P. E. (1985). Hockey success and birthdate: The relative age effect. *Journal of the Canadian Association of Health, Physical Education and Recreation, 51*, 23–28.

Cobley, S., Baker, J., Wattie, N., & McKenna, J. (2009). Annual age-grouping and athlete development. *Sports Medicine, 39*(3), 235–256.

Diaper, N. (2015). Talent identification in Paralympic Sport. *Historical and Current Aspects of National and International Dialogue in Disabled Sports 1951–2011*, 12–20.

Dutia, I., & Tweedy, S. (2021). The Paralympics strive for inclusion. But some rules unfairly exclude athletes with severe disabilities. *The Conversation.* https://theconversation.com/the-paralympics-strive-for-inclusion-but-some-rules-unfairly-exclude-athletes-with-severe-disabilities-166347

Fortin-Guichard, D., Ravensbergen, H. J. C., Krabben, K., Allen, P. M., & Mann, D.L. (1984). The Relationship Between Visual Function and Performance in Para Swimming. *Sports Medicine-Open, 8*(1), 1–18.

Grondin, S., Deshaies, P., & Nault, L.-P. (1984). Trimestre de naissance et participation au hockey et au volleyball. *La revue Québécoise de l'Activité Physique, 2*, 97–103.

Helsen, W. F., Starkes, J. L., & Van Winckel, J. (1998). The influence of relative age on success and dropout in male soccer players. *American Journal of Human Biology: The Official Journal of the Human Biology Association, 10*(6), 791–798.

International Paralympic Committee (2007). IPC Classification Code And International Standards. Retrieved September 17, 2021 from https://www.paralympic.org/sites/default/files/document/120201084329386_2008_2_Classification_Code6.pdf

International Paralympic Committee (2015). International Standard for Athlete Evaluation. Retrieved September 17, 2021 from https://www.paralympic.org/sites/default/files/document/161007092547338_Sec+ii+chapter+1_3_2_subchapter+2_International+Standard+for+Athlete+Evaluation.pdf

International Paralympic Committee. (2020). Explanatory guide to Paralympic classification. Retrieved September 17, 2021 from https://www.paralympic.org/sites/default/files/2020-10/2020_06%20Explanatory%20Guide%20to%20Classification_Summer%20Sports.pdf

International Wheelchair Rugby Federation (2021). *IWRF Classification Rules.* Etoy, Switzerland: IWRF

Kons, R., Krabben, K., Mann, D. L., & Detanico, D. (2021). Effect of vision impairment on match-related performance and technical variation in attacking moves in Paralympic judo. *Journal of Sports Sciences, 39*(sup1), 125–131.

Kons, R. L., Krabben, K., Mann, D. L., Fischer, G., & Detanico, D. (2019). The effect of vision impairment on competitive and technical-tactical performance in judo: Is the present system legitimate?. *Adapted Physical Activity Quarterly*, *36*(3), 388–398.

Krabben, K., Mashkovskiy, E., Ravensbergen, H. J. C., & Mann, D. L. (2021). May the best-sighted win? The relationship between visual function and performance in Para judo. *Journal of Sports Sciences*, *39*(sup1), 188–197.

Krabben, K., Ravensbergen, R. H., Orth, D., Fortin-Guichard, D., Savelsbergh, G. J., & Mann, D. L. (2021). Assessment of visual function and performance in Paralympic judo for athletes with vision impairment. *Optometry and Vision Science*, *98*(7), 854–863.

Krabben, K. J., van der Kamp, J., & Mann, D. L. (2018). Fight without sight: The contribution of vision to judo performance. *Psychology of Sport and Exercise*, *37*, 157–163.

Latham, K., Mann, D. L., Dolan, R., Myint, J., Timmis, M. A., Ryu, D., ... & Allen, P. M. (2021). Do visual fields need to be considered in classification criteria within visually impaired shooting?. *Journal of Sports Sciences*, *39*(sup1), 150–158.

Mann, D. L., Dehghansai, N., & Baker, J. (2017). Searching for the elusive gift: Advances in talent identification in sport. *Current Opinion in Psychology*, *16*, 128–133.

Mann, D. L., & Ravensbergen, H. J. C. (2018). International Paralympic Committee (IPC) and International Blind Sports Federation (IBSA) joint position stand on the sport-specific classification of athletes with vision impairment. *Sports Medicine*, *48*(9), 2011–2023.

Mann, D. L., Tweedy, S. M., Jackson, R. C., & Vanlandewijck, Y. C. (2021). Classifying the evidence for evidence-based classification in Paralympic sport. *Journal of Sports Sciences*, *39*(Sup 1), 1–6.

Musch, J., & Grondin, S. (2001). Unequal competition as an impediment to personal development: A review of the relative age effect in sport. *Developmental Review*, *21*(2), 147–167.

Myint, J., Latham, K., Mann, D., Gomersall, P., Wilkins, A. J., & Allen, P. M. (2016). The relationship between visual function and performance in rifle shooting for athletes with vision impairment. *BMJ Open Sport & Exercise Medicine*, *2*(1), e000080.

NOC*NSF. (2021). Future without limitations Vision of TeamNL on the paralympic sport. Retrieved January 3, 2022 from https://www.nocnsf.nl/media/5004/paralympic-vision-teamnl-nocnsf-english-version.pdf

Patterson, D. D., & Peterson, D. F. (2004). Vertical jump and leg power norms for young adults. *Measurement in Physical Education and Exercise Science*, *8*(1), 33–41.

Pérez-Torralba, A., Reina, R., Pastor-Vicedo, J. C., & González-Víllora, S. (2019). Education intervention using para-sports for athletes with high support needs to improve attitudes towards students with disabilities in Physical Education. *European Journal of Special Needs Education*, *34*(4), 455–468.

Powis, B., & Macbeth, J. L. (2020). "We know who is a cheat and who is not. But what can you do?": Athletes' perspectives on classification in visually impaired sport. *International Review for the Sociology of Sport*, *55*(5), 588–602.

Ravensbergen, H. R., Mann, D. L., & Kamper, S. J. (2016). Expert consensus statement to guide the evidence-based classification of Paralympic athletes with vision impairment: a Delphi study. *British Journal of Sports Medicine*, *50*(7), 386–391.

Spathis, J. G., Connick, M. J., Beckman, E. M., Newcombe, P. A., & Tweedy, S. M. (2015). Reliability and validity of a talent identification test battery for seated and standing Paralympic throws. *Journal of Sports Sciences*, *33*(8), 863–871.

Stalin, A., Creese, M., & Dalton, K. N. (2021). Do impairments in visual functions affect skiing performance?. *Frontiers in Neuroscience*, *15*, 648648.

Strategic Plan 2019 to 2022. (2019). International Paralympic Committee, Retrieved on September 30, 2021, from https://www.paralympic.org/sites/default/files/document/190704145051100_2019_07+IPC+Strategic+Plan_web.pdf

Tweedy, S. M., Mann D. L., & Vanlandewijck, Y. C. (2016). Research needs for the development of evidence-based systems of classification for physical, visual and intellectual impairments. In Y. C. Vanlandewijck & W. R. Thompson (Eds.) *Training and coaching of the Paralympic athlete* (pp. 122–149). IOC Press Wiley Blackwell.

Tweedy, S. M., & Vanlandewijck, Y. C. (2011). International Paralympic Committee position stand—Background and scientific principles of classification in Paralympic sport. *British Journal of Sports Medicine*, *45*(4), 259–269.

Vaeyens, R., Lenior, M., Williams, A. M., & Philippaerts, R. M. (2008). Talent identification and development programmes in sport. *Sport Medicine*, *38*(9), 703–714.

Van Biesen, D., Burns, J., Mactavish, J., Van de Vliet, P., & Vanlandewijck, Y. (2021). Conceptual model of sport-specific classification for para-athletes with intellectual impairment. *Journal of Sports Sciences*, *39*(sup1), 19–29.

Vanlandewijck, Y. C., & Thompson, W. R. (2010). *The Paralympic athlete: Handbook of sports medicine and science*. Wiley-Blackwell.

World Shooting Para Sport (2019). *Classification rules and regulations*. International Paralympic Committee. Retrieved September 17, 2021 from https://www.paralympic.org/sites/default/files/document/190207132510726_World+Shooting+Para+Sport+Classification+Rules+and+Regulations.pdf

7

STRIKING A BALANCE: PROMOTING QUANTITY AND QUALITY OF PARTICIPATION IN PARA SPORT

Alexandra J. Walters, Janet Lawson, and Amy E. Latimer-Cheung
Practitioner Commentary: Jenny Davey

Barriers to sport participation

Participation in sport is an essential component of healthy physical and social functioning (Carroll et al., 2014; Hammel et al., 2008; Labbe et al., 2019; Ryan & Deci, 2017; Sweet et al., 2021). Similarly, participation in sport at the grassroots or community level is essential to the development of elite Para athletes (Dehghansai et al., 2017). Yet, individuals with a disability face more barriers to sport participation and have fewer opportunities to participate in sport than their non-disabled counterparts (Evans et al., 2020; Orr et al., 2018; Shirazipour et al., 2020).[1] In fact, persons with disabilities are consistently reported as participating in sport and physical activity less than their non-disabled peers. For example, Sport England showed 21% of individuals living with no impairment were inactive compared with 34% of adults living with a single impairment and 51% of adults living with three or more impairments (Sport England, 2016). This participation gap is so significant the British Paralympic Association called the relatively small number Para sport participants at the community level the single biggest obstacle to future Paralympic success (Peake, 2015).

Historically, sport participation for persons with a disability has focused on increasing the number of opportunities to participate (i.e., quantity), yet the mere availability of sport opportunities does not equate to the equality of opportunities to actually engage in sport in a meaningful manner (Evans et al., 2018). Consequently, a strictly quantitative conceptualization of participation fails to capture what full and effective participation really means to athletes with a disability. Emerging models of participation propose participation in life situations such as sport must be considered in

DOI: 10.4324/9781003184430-7

terms of both quantity *and* quality (Evans et al., 2018). Prominent models of participation are described next.

Models of participation

Participation as performance

The World Health Organization's (2001) International Classification of Functioning, Disability, and Health (ICF), defines Participation[2] as the extent to which a person's 'involvement in a life situation' (p. 10) can be observed. However, many scholars have critiqued the ICF (Baylies, 2002; Heinemann et al., 2011; Pfeiffer, 2000) based on its failure to consider broader environmental and social factors (e.g., gender, family, culture) which contribute to disability (Hammell, 2015). This emphasis on observable participation implies a person can be separated from their environment for the purposes of quantifying participation (Dijkers, 2010; Hammel et al., 2008), ignores the influence of environmental and social factors on a person's capability to participate (Heinemann et al., 2011), and disregards the meaning participants attribute to their subjective participation experiences (Hammell, 2015). Instead, the ICF is said to generalize the experience of disability and participation and perpetuate medicalized understandings of disability through its focus on deficit and dysfunction at the individual level (Hammel et al., 2008). Relatedly, Ueda and Okawa (2003) suggested that focusing exclusively on quantity in participation assessments strips participation of the meaning it holds for the individual, thus reducing the utility of such a measure. Given that people view participation as an expression of their values, this is a considerable limitation.

Alternative approaches to participation

Alternative conceptualizations of participation have been proposed across numerous fields (e.g., occupational therapy, sport psychology, sociology). For example, Heinemann et al. (2011) emphasized *participation enfranchisement,* or the extent to which people feel they participate in the community in a manner that is personally valuable, as a key indicator of participation. Positive enfranchisement then relates to one's feelings of belonging to a community and freedom to participate within social networks. This viewpoint contrasts the ICF conceptualization of participation, wherein one may be highly engaged in a life activity by way of performance, yet still experience feelings of hostility and disapproval from their community. Similarly, Hammell (2015) viewed participation in terms of the capabilities approach and emphasized participation is a result of a person's (1) function or ability, (2) capability, or the combination of personal abilities, resources, and the environment, and, finally, (3) agency which is similar to autonomy. Characterizing participation in this way allows us to consider how opportunities are distributed between individuals of all abilities, thus shifting the emphasis away from disability and towards a social-ecological and subjective understanding of participation.

Hammel et al. (2008) highlighted it is seldom that people with disabilities are actively involved in the conceptualization and construction of participation assessments – such as the ICF. Thus, these types of measures prioritize the opinions of professionals over those with lived experience. Instead, Hammel et al. (2008) suggest objective measures of participation need to be flexible enough to deal with individuals' varying desires and needs and must accept that while patterns of participation may differ, they may still reflect full participation. Utilizing a participatory approach with focus groups, Hammel et al. (2008) also identified a cluster of personally meaningful themes related to participation (e.g., meaningful engagement, choice and control, and social connection, inclusion, and membership) which were not defined by a singular set of values. Rather, it was the individual's freedom to define and choose to partake in opportunities that was most important to them. Thus, the study of participation must consider diverse social relationships, groups communities, cultures, and the role the environment plays in facilitating, obstructing, and transforming participation.

The works presented so far highlight a recent focus on the *quality of participation* experiences of individuals with disabilities and targeted efforts to understand what 'full and effective participation' really means (United Nations, 2007). Support for this conceptual shift is the adoption of an alternative to the medical model of disability and deficit-based approach to assessing participation. Rather, a social-relational understanding of disability centralizes the subjective experiences of individuals with impairments while recognizing the influence of physical impairments, structural barriers, and social attitudes and discourses of disability in constructing disability (Thomas, 1999, 2004). Accordingly, disability is thought to be socially constructed, yet rooted in the bodily experience of those living with impairment.

Broadening the conceptualization of participation

Quality participation

Couched within the social-relational model of disability, Dijkers (2010) defined participation as the domain of functioning that is beyond impairment and the performance of activities. Accordingly, Dijkers (2010) suggested the complex relationship between the individual and society, as well as biological and social standards of normality are critical components in defining and operationalizing the concept of participation. Despite the appreciation of a qualitative view of participation, differing taxonomies from independent investigations remain problematic for decision-makers and service providers who aim to foster meaningful participation experiences, deliver programs, and provide services for persons with a disability. Specifically, it is difficult for stakeholders to determine a collective path for meaningful participation without a shared taxonomy to underpin their efforts.

Most recently addressing this gap in the literature, Martin Ginis et al. (2017) extended our understanding of these subjective aspects of participation by advancing a holistic conceptualization of participation for persons with physical disabilities, which included cross-discipline recommendations. Through a rigorous systematic configurative review of participation literature, Martin Ginis et al. (2017) concluded that participation quality is made up of an individual's positive subjective perception of their acute, in-the-moment experiences (herein labeled, quality experiences). Quality experiences feature one or more of the following experiential elements: belongingness, autonomy, challenge, engagement, mastery, and meaning (see Figure 7.1). Importantly, quality experiences are the result of a dynamic interplay between experiential elements. While individuals may vary in the amount they value each element, all participants should have the opportunity to satisfy each of the six elements. Repeated exposure over time to experiential elements is said to result in quality participation (Evans et al., 2018). Furthermore, these experiential elements are cross-cutting such that they apply across life domains including mobility, employment, sport and exercise (Caron et al., 2019).

Quality participation in Para sport

Evans et al. (2018) operationalized Martin Ginis et al.'s (2017) conceptualization of participation within Para sport contexts resulting in the development of the Quality Parasport Participation Framework (*QPPF*).

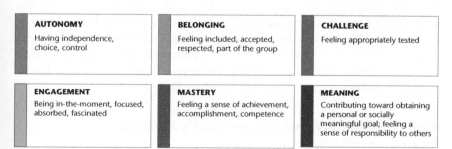

AUTONOMY	BELONGING	CHALLENGE
Having independence, choice, control	Feeling included, accepted, respected, part of the group	Feeling appropriately tested
ENGAGEMENT	**MASTERY**	**MEANING**
Being in-the-moment, focused, absorbed, fascinated	Feeling a sense of achievement, accomplishment, competence	Contributing toward obtaining a personal or socially meaningful goal; feeling a sense of responsibility to others

FIGURE 7.1 Elements of a quality experience (Canadian Disability Participation Project, 2018)

Central to the QPPF are the six elements of quality experience. Extending from there, the QPPF outlines 25 conditions (i.e., aspects such as rules, facilities, normative beliefs, and policies) across sport activities, the physical environment, and the social environment which support quality experiences (see Evans et al. [2018] for the full list of conditions). These conditions were derived from research evidence and a rigorous process of stakeholder feedback.

For example, Shirazipour et al. (2020) conducted a systematic review of program environments, which fosters elements of quality participation. These included group-based programming, and knowledgeable leaders. Evidence provided links between group composition fostering feelings of *belongingness* and *mastery* through groups composition (i.e., small, or large groups, similarity or difference in ability represented within a group). Leadership of coaches and instructors was identified as a factor influencing *mastery* and *autonomy,* especially instructors with disability-specific knowledge, who ensured participants felt safe and that the program would suit their needs (Shirazipour, 2020). In turn, athletes felt empowered to continue participating in sport. Notably, these conditions were not facilitators of quality experiences themselves, rather they were fundamental to quality experiences.

Of promise, emerging research corroborates the conditions for fostering the experiential elements. A recent evaluation of physical activity programs for persons with a disability described groups as providing participants with a sense of social connection (Sweet et al., 2021). An exploration of the physical activity experiences of youth emphasized the importance of participating with peers of similar impairments or abilities to foster meaningful social relationships, peer support, and mentorship (i.e., *belongingness*; Orr et al., 2020; Orr et al., 2018).

In describing the QPFF, Evans et al. identified the hierarchy of the Framework as important – wherein prior to an athlete experiencing quality participation, a minimum standard (i.e., a threshold) of physical, social, and program conditions must be met. For example, at an absolute minimum, the sport venue must be accessible (e.g., have ramps, accessible bathrooms) to afford the athlete opportunity to participate and experience the quality elements. Once this threshold is met, it is the personally meaningful and ever-changing combination of experiential elements that constitute an athlete's subjective feeling of quality participation (see Figure 7.2).

A common language within the Quality Participation Parasport Framework

Although Martin Ginis et al.'s (2017) conceptualization of quality participation and Evans et al.'s (2018) QPPF were developed with and for the

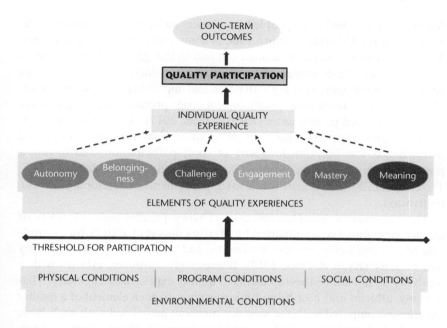

FIGURE 7.2 The Quality Parasport Participation Framework (adapted from Evans et al., 2018)

disability community using disability-focused research evidence, many of the key concepts are proving universal. Notably, the six elements of a quality experience align with various constructs in established theories of human behavior and well-being. This alignment is a strength. The similarities in the frameworks, despite variation in methods of development and target audience, lend mutual validity highlighting critical components of positive or quality experience. Practitioners and researchers can draw from existing theoretical knowledge to begin to explore and tailor new potential intervention strategies for fostering quality experience. The complementarity of the QPPF with three theories or frameworks applied in non-disabled sport are considered next.

Self-Determination Theory

Self-Determination Theory is a prominent psychological theory that has been applied to explain athletes' motivations to participate in sport (Ryan & Deci, 2017; Teixeira et al., 2012). Positing that autonomy, relatedness, and competence make up humans' three basic psychological needs, Self-Determination Theory suggests humans seek out and engage in opportunities to satisfy these needs to optimize well-being (i.e., need satisfaction; Ryan & Deci, 2017).

Autonomy is satisfied when people have choices and a sense of independence. Relatedness is satisfied by feeling a sense of community and relating to others. And competence is satisfied through optimal challenge and feelings of mastery. Sport-specific examples of need satisfaction include making choices about training designs, working with peers, and improving one's performance. Meeting athletes' three basic psychological needs promotes intrinsic motivation and sustained participation (Ryan & Deci, 2017). As intrinsically motivated athletes experience more positive sport outcomes (e.g., improved performance, less burnout, longevity of sport participation, and having a positive influence on team morale; Cheon et al., 2015; Ryan & Deci, 2017; Teixeira et al., 2012), it is worthwhile to support athletes in developing intrinsic motivation.

The premises of Self-Determination Theory parallel some elements of quality experiences conceptualized by Martin Ginis et al. (2017), for example relatedness and belongingness, autonomy and autonomy, and competency and mastery (Ryan & Deci, 2017). Interestingly, however, athletes with a disability do not define these elements of quality experiences singularly. That is to say, athletes may ascribe multiple meanings to each element of a quality experience compared with the singular meaning associated with each basic psychological needs described in Self-Determination Theory. For example, Allan et al. (2018) reported belongingness as a central component of three distinct participation narratives. Belongingness was associated with social status in the performance narrative, social acceptance in the relational narrative, and a sense of community in the discovery narrative. Though each athlete's definition was associated with the broader experiential element of belongingness, the individual and contextually based description of what belongingness meant to each athlete indicates a nuanced perspective of belongingness which is unique to Para sport contexts. Thus, the QPPF offers novel, disability-specific to compliment Self-Determination Theory.

Personal Assets Framework

The QPPF as a whole also carries many similarities to the Personal Assets Framework used in youth sport settings (Côté et al., 2014). The development of the Personal Assets Framework was informed by positive youth development research and developmental systems theories (Côté et al., 2020). It suggests an appropriate setting, quality social dynamics, and personal engagement interact over time (e.g., a sport season or quadrennial between World Championships or Olympic Games) to foster immediate, short-term, and long-term developmental outcomes in athletes (Côté et al., 2020). Within this framework, *appropriate setting* refers to the physical and competitive context and includes micro- and macro-environments. For example, the playing field, the club/organizational structure, and the community structure.

This parallels conditions of the physical environment described by Evans et al. (2018). *Quality social dynamics* refers to the highly social nature of sport, wherein interactions with teammates, coaches, spectators, and others, can enhance or detract from the experience quality (Bruner, et al., 2020). This factor encompasses nested levels beginning with interpersonal relationships, team dynamics, and ending with the broader social environment and reflects the social environment described by Evans et al. (2018). Lastly, *personal engagement in activities* includes the sport of interest, and complementary physical and non-sport related activities, all of which contribute to the achievement of long-term positive developmental outcomes (Côté et al., 2020). Here, activities such as practice and game play echo conditions of the sport activity included in the QPPF.

Transformational leadership

Within the QPPF, several leadership behaviors are identified as strategies for fostering the quality elements (see Figure 7.2). Specifically, autonomy-supportive coaching practices, such as including positive verbal feedback, highlighting opportunities for choice, and encouraging athletes to take initiative (Cheon et al., 2015; Evans et al., 2020; Orr et al., 2018; Ryan & Deci, 2017), may foster athletes' intrinsic motivation to participate in sport. This may further support quality experiences through their influence on team cohesion, player satisfaction, and team outcomes (Cheon et al., 2015; Ryan & Deci, 2017). A coaching style that shows promise in this regard is transformational coaching. Based in transformational leadership, this type of coaching is person-centered and characterized by coaches encouraging and inspiring athletes to achieve positive outcomes and to become leaders by enacting *idealized influence* (i.e., gaining followers' respect by acting as a positive role model), *inspirational motivation* (i.e., inspiring followers through a collective vision), *intellectual stimulation* (i.e., empowering followers to contribute new ideas), and *individualized consideration* (i.e., displaying genuine care and concern for followers; Bass & Riggio, 2006).

Recognizing the potential for transformational leadership as a means of fostering the experiential elements of quality participation, Chen (2020) pilot tested a transformational coaching workshop tailored for Para sport coaches. The workshop was meticulously tailored with themes from a series of evidence-based disability-focused narrative stories and was shown to significantly increase coaches' perceived capability and opportunity to demonstrate transformational coaching, as well as their perceived capability to facilitate quality experiences for athletes. This study highlights the potential for practitioners and researchers to use and tailor frameworks complimentary to the QPPF for intervention development.

Outcomes of quality experiences

Collection of data definitively establishing the outcomes of quality experience is currently underway. Given the compatibility of the QPPF with other theories and frameworks, we hypothesize athletes with disabilities experience similar outcomes from engaging in quality experiences as their non-disabled peers who are involved in an appropriate sport setting, experience quality social dynamics, and have their needs met and engaged through personally meaningful activities. According to the Personal Assets Framework, participation in non-disabled sport is said to result in the development of confidence (i.e., a positive sense of overall self-worth), competence (i.e., sport-specific skills and knowledge as well as physical fitness), connection (i.e., positive relationships with people inside and outside of sport), and character (i.e., integrity and respect for the sport) over the short-term and continued participation, personal development, and performance improvement long-term (Côté et al., 2020). These positive outcomes are consistent with the reported outcomes of quality experiences. For example, physical activity programs for military veterans have resulted in short-term outcomes such as enjoyment, fostered by positive group environments and coach support (Shirazipour & Latimer-Cheung, 2016), which is representative of connection as described by Côté and Gilbert (2009). Moreover, Shirazipour and Latimer-Cheung (2016) found the same programs facilitate mental healing and pride as a result of positive relationships with family and peers, goal achievement, and finding meaning in sport over the long-term, demonstrating competence and confidence as described by Côté and Gilbert (2009).

Turnnidge et al. (2012) found athletes participating in an exceptional Para Swimming program at the provincial through to international levels of competition experienced redefined capabilities, an affirmed sense of self, strengthened social connection, and enhanced acceptance (of theirs and others' disabilities). These outcomes, which demonstrate the relevance of quality experiences across the developmental continuum, were facilitated by various aspects of the social environment, including positive coach-athlete relationships and peer interactions. This evidence further supports the assertion that coaches are important social agents within sport who have a considerable impact on athletes' well-being (Horn, 2008), and align with more recent literature which indicates coaches' interpersonal behaviors contribute to the development of athlete outcomes in sport (Allan et al., 2019).

Practical recommendations for facilitating quality participation

A tangible tool to complement the QPPF, the Blueprint for Building Quality Participation in Sport for Children, Youth, and Adults with a Disability is available as a checklist and audit tool to sports program builders to ensure key components of quality participation are reflected in their program's delivery (Canadian Disability Participation Project, 2018). For brevity, the final section of this chapter will highlight some of the recommendations shared by Blueprint that have been discussed in this chapter, and that are specific to (1) coaches and (2) disability sports organizations. While the tips below do not constitute an exhaustive list, a complete list of practical strategies for additional stakeholders in an athlete's network can be found elsewhere (see Canadian Disbality Participation Project, 2018).

Coaches

Through the social environment, coaches can exert a tremendous amount of influence on an athlete's participation experience (Jeanes et al., 2014; Orr et al., 2020; Ryan & Deci, 2017) and their attitudes towards others. Social support and social processes have knock-on effects on the athlete's self-concept, affect, and emotion (Martin Ginis et al., 2016). Allan et al. (2019) demonstrated coaches are a significant determinant of athlete outcomes in Para sport contexts. Specifically, Allan et al. (2019) clarified coaches can positively influence athletes' experiences by enacting consideration, collaboration, and professionalism. Consideration is a reflective process wherein the coach anticipates, understands, and reflects on athletes' needs while recognizing and situating their own biases and assumptions relating to sport and disability. Collaboration is mutual learning and development characterized by shared beliefs, values, and expectations. Professionalism refers to the coach's competency or specialized knowledge and skill derived from relevant experience. Meanwhile, coaches were also shown to negatively influence athletes' experiences when they act in a prejudicial manner. Prejudicial actions included demonstrating oppressive attitudes or behaviors resulting from a lack of knowledge and experience as well as stereotypical understandings of disability and Para sport.

Practically, Paralympic coaches who provide their athletes with choice and initiative have been shown to facilitate feelings of autonomy and engagement in elite sport (Banack et al., 2011; Cheon et al., 2015). Additionally, coaches who utilize simple, practical strategies to foster quality experiences, such as organizing friendly inter-squad competitions, celebrating athletes' successes via social media, and establishing peer-mentorship opportunities, have successfully fostered elements of challenge and mastery, resulting in quality experiences for athletes (Fong et al., 2020). It is critical coaches recognize their role in their athlete's participation experience, and then adopt evidence-based coaching strategies that can facilitate a social environment for quality participation to be experienced by athletes with an impairment. Such strategies may include:

1. Adopting an autonomy-support coaching style (Cheon et al., 2015; Evans et al., 2020; Ryan & Deci, 2017). This includes a focus on providing positive verbal feedback, highlighting opportunities for improvement, providing choice, being responsive to athletes' ideas and questions, minimizing demands, encouraging leadership, and allowing opportunities for personal choice.
2. Focusing on outcomes such as enjoyment and fun, rather than winning or performance (Orr et al., 2020). This can be as simple as providing athletes with the choice of music during practice drills.
3. Fostering a sense of team and group cohesion by giving roles to team members (Evans et al., 2020; Orr et al., 2020). This will help each member feel like they are contributing to a meaningful goal. Some roles can include a team captain, a social events leader, or an equipment holder.
4. Seeking opportunities to improve disability-specific knowledge and coaching skills (Bruno et al., 2021).
5. Appreciating the uniqueness of each athlete, and working with them individually when possible (Evans et al., 2020; Shirazipour et al., 2020). Each athlete experiences quality participation in their own way and may value different experiential elements are different times (Evans et al., 2018).
6. Checking-in with athletes often to ensure they are feeling supported in their athletic endeavours (Bruno et al., in preparation; Sweet et al., 2021).

Disability sports organizations

Disability sports organizations directly influence the program environment. Organizations should, therefore, begin by adapting their program vision and mission to align with the principles of quality participation. Ways organizations can facilitate quality participation are to:

1. Prioritize time for vision and mission planning at the start of each sports season. Seek opportunities for program evaluation, which can highlight opportunities for improvement (Bruno et al., in preparation; Orr et al., 2020; Shirazipour et al., 2020).
2. Provide sports programs that offer a variety of entry levels. This will help athletes choose a level that is appropriate to their abilities and form lasting relationships with similar peers (Evans et al., 2020; Evans et al., 2018; Orr et al., 2018).
3. Be mindful of group size – especially in youth sport. A smaller ratio of athletes to coaches is preferable to teams that have athletes with a variety of abilities (Orr et al., 2020).
4. Recognize the value of listening to the athletes' motivations when joining a sport program. For example, at registration ask them what

they hope to achieve from their participation (e.g., make friends, gain skills; Bruno et al., in preparation; Evans et al., 2020).

5. Offer and encourage coach training opportunities to improve their disability-specific knowledge (Bruno et al., in preparation).
6. Form alliances with other disability sport organizations. This will manage the flow of information between organizations, and work towards collective aims of providing quality Para sport programs for athletes (Konoval et al., 2019; Martin Ginis et al., 2016).

Concluding thoughts

Through reading this chapter you should have developed a fulsome understanding of the concept of quality participation in Para sport. You should be aware of the limitations of the common conceptualizations of participation focused exclusively on quantity. Namely, that these conceptualizations fail to wholly capture full and effective participation in the Para sport context. Building on this, the concept of quality participation and the Quality Participation Parasport Framework (QPPF) were introduced as alternative ways of considering participation for athletes with disabilities. Additionally, various ways in which quality participation can be facilitated throughout an athlete's development were presented, alongside commonalities and limitations of other frameworks relevant to disability, participation, and athletic development (e.g., International Classification of Functioning, Disability, and Health; Self-Determination Theory; Personal Assets Framework). Through this, you should have learned how stakeholders can facilitate quality experiences for athletes and, ultimately, foster quality participation and support athlete development. In sum, through reading this chapter, you should now be familiar with various models of participation and have an understanding of how quality participation experiences can be facilitated in a variety of sport contexts.

Practitioner commentary

The concept in the chapter title of 'striking a balance' is so important when considering Para sport systems. At times, I think Para sport whittles itself into binary, or at least compartmentalized, ways of thinking and organizing – it's either quality *or* quantity of experience; it's integrated *or* segregated programming; it might be *this* Classification, but not others. This tendency can be so limiting, and can impede individuals' autonomy, choice, and belonging, especially earlier in the sport journey.

For example, there is often a sort of mantra that integration (i.e., Para sport delivery nested within nondisabled settings, or led by non-Para organizations) is the ultimate indicator of a fully accessible sport system.

There can be a view that integrated sport organizations or experiences will automatically translate to appropriate, equitable, and positive experiences. While conceptually well-intended, in reality that push sometimes results in a *same same same* mentality – as in, same rules, same planning, same coaching, etc., for everyone no matter their interests, experiences, disability (ies), or other individual characteristics. These blanket approaches run contrary to the philosophy and components of quality participation. Participants may feel they have less choice in their experiences, or they might struggle to access the right level of challenge in this rigid environment. The *same same same* style may certainly work for a few individuals. However, what I see and hear in my daily work is that more customized and nuanced approaches, perhaps a blend of integrated and segregated experiences so that participants can sample and find the right fit, are often preferred and lead to more consistently positive experiences.

Additionally, the urgency for increasing the number of participants still looms large at all levels. I have seen grassroots clubs that strive to churn out participation rates on par with their non-Para counterparts because they believe the numbers will elevate their worth in the eyes of funders (sadly, they are sometimes correct). So, they rush to gather as many volunteers as possible to support the greatest number of athletes every season, but at the expense of taking the time to train volunteers effectively or to listen to athlete needs. The result is an impressive number on the surface, but often less meaningful – or worse, less safe, or even harmful – experiences for all involved. There are excellent organizations and individuals leading thoughtful, tailored, participant-centered programming; unfortunately, they sometimes get shut out of the funding, resource, and recognition race for being bold enough to focus on quality over quantity.

Participants arrive at Para sport with such a vast spectrum of experiences, needs, goals, and interests. That's a strength – we have a lot to learn from each other, and this diversity contributes to a rich and exciting environment. I would love to see the system keep evolving to embrace that diversity further, and be comfortable with doing things differently in Para, so that we better support each person's unique needs to access positive experiences, and ultimately, quality participation.

Notes

1 This chapter speaks to athletes with a disability generally, including diverse age groups and disability types. Much of the literature speaks to research with adults with a physical disability; however, the findings and recommendations are not exclusive to this subgroup.
2 Participation denoted with a capital (i.e., Participation), as well as Participation Restrictions, and Performance refer to the ICF taxonomy. When used without capitalization, the terms refer to these concepts more broadly.

References

Allan, V., Evans, B. M., Latimer-Cheung, A. E., & Côté, J. (2019). From the athletes' perspective: A social-relational understanding of how coaches shape the disability sport experience. *Journal of Applied Sport Psychology, 32*, 546–564.

Allan, V., Smith, B., Côté, J., Martin Ginis, K. A., & Latimer-Cheung, A. E. (2018). Narratives of participation among individuals with physical disabilities: A life-course analysis of athletes' experiences and development in parasport. *Psychology of Sport and Exercise, 37*, 170–178.

Banack, H. R., Sabiston, C. M., & Bloom, G. A. (2011). Coach autonomy support, basic need satisfaction and intrinsic motivation of Paralympic athletes. *Research Quarterly for Exercise and Sport, 82*, 722–730.

Bass, B. M., & Riggio, R. E. (2006). *Transformational leadership* (2nd ed.). New York, NY: Psychology Press.

Baylies, C. (2002). Disability and the notion of human development: Questions of rights and capabilities. *Disability and Society, 17*, 725–739.

Bruner, M. W., Eys, M. A., & Martin, L. J. (2020). *The power of groups in youth sport*. London, UK: Elsevier.

Bruno, N., Tomasone, J. R., Arbour-Nicitopoulos, K., Davies, T., Borer, R., & Latimer-Cheung, A. E. (2021). Utilizing knowledge translation to enhance quality participation in recreational sport programming for children with intellectual and developmental disabilities. Manuscript in preparation.

Canadian Disability Participation Project. (2018). *A blueprint for building quality participation in sport for children, youth, and adults with a disability*. Kelowna, BC: University of British Columbia.

Caron, J. G., Martin Ginis, K. A., Rocchi, M., & Sweet, S. N. (2019). Development of the measure of experiential aspects of participation for people with physical disabilities. *Archives of Physical Medicine and Rehabilitation, 100*(1), 67–77.

Carroll, D. D., Courtney-Long, E. A., Stevens, A. C., Sloan, M. L., Lullo, C., Visser, S. N., Fox, M. H., Armour, B. S., Campbell, V. A., Brown, D. R., Dorn, J. M., & Centers for Disease Control and Prevetion. (2014). Vital signs: Disability and physical activity-United States, 2009–2012. *Morbidity and Mortality Weekly Report, 63*(18), 407–413.

Chen, J. (2020). Assessing the impact and delivery of the transformational coaching workshop in Para sport. Master's thesis, Queen's University. ProQuest. Retrieved from https://www.proquest.com/openview/6317e3b4a9e0b613be56b0cbb6a693a2/1.pdf?pq-origsite=gscholar&cbl=18750&diss=y

Cheon, S. H., Reeve, J., Lee, J., & Lee, Y. (2015). Giving and receiving autonomy support in a high-stakes sport context: A field-based experiment during the 2012 London Paralympic Games. *Psychology of Sport and Exercise, 19*, 59–69.

Côté, J., & Gilbert, W. (2009). An integrative definition of coaching effectiveness and expertise. *International Journal of Sports Science and Coaching, 4*, 307–323.

Côté, J., Turnnidge, J., & Evans, M. B. (2014). The dynamic process of development through sport. *Kinesiologica Slovenica: Scientific Journal on Sport, 20*, 14–26.

Côté, J., Turnnidge, J., Murata, A., McGuire, C., & Martin, L. (2020). Youth sport research: Describing the integrated dynamics elements of the Personal Assets Framework. *International Journal of Sport Psychology, 51*(6), 562–578.

Dehghansai, N., Lemez, S., Wattie, N., & Baker, J. (2017). A systematic review of influences on development of athletes with disabilities. *Adapted Physical Activity Quarterly, 34*(1), 72–90.

Dijkers, M. P. (2010). Issues in the conceptualization and measurement of participation: An overview. *Archives of Physical Medicine and Rehabilitation, 91*(9 Suppl), S5–S16.

Evans, M. B., Graupensperger, S., & Arbour-Nicitopoulos, K. P. (2020). Peer groups in disbality sport. In Bruner. M., Eys. M., & Martin. L. (Eds.), *The power of groups in youth sport* (pp. 303–326). Academic Press.

Evans, M. B., Shirazipour, C. H., Allan, V., Zanhour, M., Sweet, S. N., Martin Ginis, K. A., & Latimer-Cheung, A. E. (2018). Integrating insights from the parasport community to understand optimal experiences: The Quality Parasport Participation Framework. *Psychology of Sport and Exercise, 37*, 79–90.

Fong, A. J., Saxton, H. R., Kauffeldt, K. D., Sabiston C.M., & Tomasone, J. R. (2020). "We're all in the same boat together": Exploring quality participation strategies in dragon boat teams for breast cancer survivors. *Disability and Rehabilitation, 43*(21), 3078–3089.

Hammel, J., Magasi, S., Heinemann, A., Whiteneck, G., Bogner, J., & Rodriguez, E. (2008). What does participation mean? An insider perspective from people with disabilities. *Disability and Rehabilitation, 30*(19), 1445–1460.

Hammell, K. W. (2015). Quality of life, participation and occupational rights: A capabilities perspective. *Australian Occupational Therapy Journal, 62*(2), 78–85.

Heinemann, A. W., Lai, J. S., Magasi, S., Hammel, J., Corrigan, J. D., Bogner, J. A., & Whiteneck, G. G. (2011). Measuring participation enfranchisement. *Archives of Physical Medical and Rehabilitation, 92*(4), 564–571.

Horn, T. S. (2008). Coaching effectiveness in the sport domain. In T. S. Horn (Ed.), *Advances in sport psychology* (3rd ed., pp. 239–267). Champaign, IL: Human Kinetics.

Jeanes, R., Magee, J., & O'Connor, J. (2014). Through Coaching: Examining a Socio-ecological Approach to Sports Coaching. In B. Wattchow, R. Jeanes, L. Alfrey, T. Brown, A. Cutter-Mackenzie, & J. O'Connor (Eds.), *The socio-ecological educator: A 21st century renewal of physical, health, environment and outdoor education* (pp. 89–107). Springer Netherlands.

Konoval, T., Leo, J., & Ferguson, J. (2019). *Becoming Para ready: A resource to help club and school athletics programs suport more effective integration.* Steward Centre for Personal & Physical Acheivement.

Labbe, D., Miller, W. C., & Ng, R. (2019). Participating more, participating better: Health benefits of adaptive leisure for people with disabilities. *Disabilty Health Journal, 12*(2), 287–295.

Martin Ginis, K. A., Evans, M. B., Mortenson, W. B., & Noreau, L. (2017). Broadening the conceptualization of participation of persons with physical disabilities: A configurative review and recommendations. *Archives of Physical Medicine and Rehabilitation, 98*(2), 395–402.

Martin Ginis, K. A., Ma, J. K., Latimer-Cheung, A. E., & Rimmer, J. H. (2016). A systematic review of review articles addressing factors related to physical activity participation among children and adults with physical disabilities. *Health Psychology Review, 10*(4), 478–494.

Orr, K., Evans, M. B., Tamminen, K. A., & Arbour-Nicitopoulos, K. P. (2020). A scoping review of recreational sport programs for disabled emerging adults. *Research Quarterly for Exercise and Sport, 91*(1), 142–157.

Orr, K., Tamminen, K. A., Sweet, S. N., Tomasone, J. R., & Arbour-Nicitopoulos, K. P. (2018). "I've had bad experiences with team sport": Sport participation, peer need-thwarting, and need-supporting behaviors among youth identifying with physical disability. *Adapted Physical Activity Quartery, 35*(1), 36–56.

Peake, R. (2015). *International Sporting Success Factors for United Kingdom Paralympic Athletes.* Presentation at the 2015 World Congress on Elite Sport Policy, Melbourne.

Pfeiffer, D. (2000). The devils are in the details: The ICIDH2 and the disability movement. *Disability and Society, 15,* 1079–1082.

Ryan, R. M., & Deci, E. L. (2017). Sport, physical activity, and physical education. In Ryan, R. M. & Deci, E. L. (Eds.), *Self-determination theory: Basic psychological needs in motivation, development, and wellness* (pp. 481–507). Guilfod.

Shirazipour, C. H., Evans, M. B., Leo, J., Lithopoulos, A., Martin Ginis, K. A., & Latimer-Cheung, A. E. (2020). Program conditions that foster quality physical activity participation experiences for people with a physical disability: A systematic review. *Disability and Rehabilitation, 42*(2), 147–155.

Shirazipour, C. H., & Latimer-Cheung, A. E. (2016). Exploring the parasport pathways of military veterans with a physical disability. *Journal of Sport and Exercise Psychology, 38*(S1), S255.

Smith, L., Wedgwood, N., Llewellyn, G., & Shuttleworth, R. (2015). Sport in the lives of people with intellectual disabilities: Negotiating disability, identity, and belonging. *Journal of Sport Development, 3*(5), 1–10.

Sport England. (2016). *Active lives survey (year 1 report).* Sport England. https://www.sportengland.org/media/11498/active-lives-survey-yr-1-report.pdf

Sweet, S. N., Shi, Z., Rocchi, M., Ramsay, J., Page, V., Lamontagne, M. E., & Gainforth, H. L. (2021). Longitudinal examination of leisure-time physical activity (LTPA), participation, and social inclusion upon joining a community-based ltpa program for adults with physical disabilities. *Archives of Physical Medicine and Rehabilitation, 102*(9), 1746–1754.

Teixeira, P. J., Carraça, E. V., Markland, D., Silva, M. N., & Ryan, R. M. (2012). Exercise, physical activity, and self-determination theory: A systematic review. *International Journal of Behavioral Nutrition and Physical Activity, 9*(1), 78.

Thomas, C. (1999). *Female forms: Experiencing and understanding disability.* Oxfordshire: Open University Press.

Thomas, C. (2004). Rescuing a social relational understanding of disability. *Scandinavian Journal of Disability Research, 6,* 22–36.

Turnnidge, J., Vierimaa, M., & Côté, J. (2012). An in-depth investigation of a model sport program for athletes with a physical disability. *Psychology, 3*(12), 1131.

Ueda, S. & Okawa, Y. (2003). The subjective dimension of functioning and disability: What is it and what is it for? *Disability and Rehabilitation, 25,* 596–601.

United Nations. (2007). *Convention on the Rights of Persons with Disabilities.* Geneva: United Nations.

World Health Organization. (2001). *International Classification of Functionning, Disablity and Health (ICF).* Geneva: World Health Organization.

8

THE ROLE OF SKILL ACQUISITION IN COACH AND ATHLETE DEVELOPMENT IN PARALYMPIC SPORT

Ross A. Pinder, Daniel Powell, Stephen Hadlow, and Georgia Askew
Practitioner Commentary: Raôul R. D. Oudejans

Introduction

Practical and theoretical frameworks centred around skill acquisition (SA) aim to provide opportunities and techniques to enhance athletes' learning. The role of the SA specialist is to work alongside athletes and coaches to support the development and co-creation of effective learning environments (Dehghansai et al., 2020a). Despite the recent emergence of a body of work aimed at understanding how coaches develop in Para sport (see Townsend et al., 2021 for a critical review), a disconnect between contemporary research in skill acquisition and coaching practice is often observed in sports, including in Paralympic contexts. Several researchers have highlighted reasons for this, including lack of access to suitable development opportunities (McMaster et al., 2012), limited mechanisms for knowledge translation (Stodter & Cushion, 2019), reliance on tradition, intuition, or custodial approaches (Moy et al., 2016), and/or decontextualised research which fails to capture the rationale underpinning coaches' learning designs (Kearney et al., 2018). Considering the nuances associated with athletes' impairments and the need for an individualized approach, this disconnect has important implications for Para athlete development, as coaches may not be adequately equipped to optimise skill learning. Additionally, there is relatively little research conducted in Para sport, with concerns such as homogeneity of participants and experimental control creating barriers for publishing and translating key insights. The reality is, there is limited knowledge on the extent to which the existing research transfers to varying populations and impairment types in Para sport contexts. To highlight this concern, a recent systematic review (Dehghansai

DOI: 10.4324/9781003184430-8

et al., 2017) identified a single empirical study which had captured a learning intervention with a Paralympic (i.e., elite) cohort over a concerted period of time (see Oudejans et al., 2012). To address some of these issues, practitioners have highlighted the need for more research exploring coaches' experiential knowledge (Greenwood et al., 2014), seeking creative ways of bridging gaps between theoretical and empirical research and coaching practice (Powell et al., 2021). Furthermore, recent moves to embed SA practitioners in daily performance environments (DPEs), allows for better insight into current practices and a means to enhance talent development pathways. While calls for more embedded coach support are not new, these Para sport contexts (e.g., Australia) may in fact be a frontrunner in translation of knowledge for coach and athlete development, with support methods tailored towards how coaches prefer to learn and develop knowledge (Fairhurst et al., 2017).

In this chapter, we highlight some of the ways applied SA support and research programs can enhance coach and athlete development in Para sport through i) identifying and addressing gaps between the scientific literature and current coaching practice, ii) empirical and applied interventions, and iii) the SA specialist supporting iterative co-creation in DPEs. While we acknowledge that a long-term approach could see these roles having a greater and more sustainable impact earlier in talent development pathways (also see Pinder et al., 2020), we limit our focus on this chapter to initial insights gained in elite Paralympic contexts in Great Britain and Australia.

I. Identifying and addressing the gaps between research and coaching practice

While there may be similarities with training methods and session designs across non-disabled and Para sport contexts, there are inherent differences between contexts including lower levels of resourcing for sport science support (Paulson & Goosey-Tolfrey, 2017). In many disciplines, including SA, support is typically leveraged through post-graduate research programs and collaborative partnerships between National bodies and Universities. While this is a creative use of resources, it can limit the flexibility and scope of support. In this chapter, we provide examples of embedded research partnerships (e.g., Case study one), and 'pooled' resources for SA support through a National Paralympic Committee (NPC). Regardless of the approach, for optimal coach and athlete support, individual (i.e., needs, impairment) and environmental (i.e., resources) constraints should be considered, which are often more extreme in Para sport contexts (Fairhurst et al., 2017; Townsend et al., 2021); essentially, research and applied support needs to embrace and understand the nonlinear nature of both coach and athlete development.

One strategy taken in SA is to better understand the knowledge and rationale underpinning coaching approaches. For example, Powell and colleagues (2021) took a mixed-methods approach and observed coaching sessions delivered by nine senior coaches from the British Para Swimming (BPS) World Class Programme, with follow up semi-structured interviews. Sessions provided quantitative data on the current (albeit snapshot) practices of coaches in relation to recommendations from some prominent lines of inquiry in SA, including their approach to focus of attention (FOA), contextual interference (CI or variability), and implicit and explicit learning strategies. Follow up interviews explored the rationale behind the structure and content of the sessions. This research served to highlight gaps between existing research and current practice to provide context for the SA specialist to begin to impact learning design. We explore how this evolved in detail in Case study one.

Case study I – Exploring and addressing gaps between SA research and applied practice in the British Para swimming (BPS) World Class Programme

The research program at BPS was created in recognition that something was missing between the biomechanical analysis of a swimmer's technique, and the application of coaching skills to implement any recommended changes. A persistent challenge discussed by coaches was in getting new skills to 'stick'. To work effectively with the coaches, it was important to first understand their current approaches to learning, and how the techniques they were adopting mapped onto current scientific recommendations.

The SA specialist began by immersing himself in the DPE at the National Performance Centre, familiarising themselves with training methods, the language of the sport, and most importantly building relationships with the coaches, athletes, and support staff. The next step involved a more formal analysis of coaching, examining practices relative to some of the established principles of SA theory. Coaching sessions across the program were observed, and interviews served to shed light on the knowledge and rationale underpinning the approaches. This research (see Powell et al., 2021) helped lay the foundations for work with the coaches in the lead up to the Tokyo 2020 Paralympic Games.

It was apparent from early discussions that the coaches had limited knowledge of key SA concepts. Furthermore, the coaches, who had all come from backgrounds in non-disabled sport, did not report following any formal guidance with regards to the coaching of Para athletes. In line with previous findings (Cregan et al., 2007; Fairhurst et al., 2017), coaches favoured informal learning opportunities for development (e.g., trial and error; observing or communicating with other coaches). As such, they had developed their own practice-informed theories of how to coach based on what had worked for them.

In relation to language, coaches were observed using cues which predominantly focused athletes' attention internally towards component parts of the body movement (e.g., 'pull your hands back'), as opposed to cues which focused attention externally towards movement effects (e.g., 'push the water back'), indicating practices may be sub-optimal for the acquisition of skills (Wulf, 2013). Interestingly, this was not the case during the coaching of start and turn skills, where coaches emphasised a more external focus (see Figure 8.1) and adopted a range of alternative cues that research suggests better facilitate athlete learning, including both holistic cues (Mullen et al., 2015) and analogies (Masters et al., 2019). However, the coaches reported little awareness of their use of such cues, and/or did not appear to view them as significant. On occasions when coaches were observed using cues such as analogies or external focus outside of starts and turns, they were typically used alongside multiple other (predominantly internal) cues, making it difficult to detect an athlete's subsequent focus. In one typical example, a coach was observed using two analogies during one set of freestyle drill instructions alongside 22 other focus cues within two minutes of dialogue. These observations and insights provided a framework for discussions and exploring new approaches with the coaches. For instance, the SA specialist was able to use the coaches' own analogies (e.g., 'imagine the wall is red hot and kick off as quickly as possible') to describe how subsequent learning benefits operate

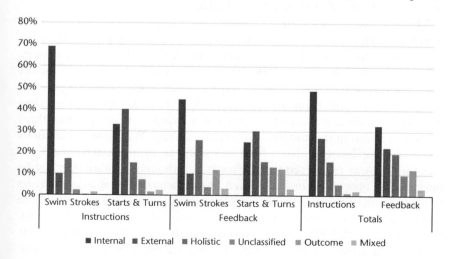

FIGURE 8.1 Coaches' use of cues during instructions and feedback for i) swim strokes and ii) starts and turns practices

as a function of reducing the athletes' reliance on working memory processes during practice (i.e., by allowing athletes to label movement instructions symbolically). Subsequently, through a collaborative approach, new verbal cues were explored (e.g., in the butterfly: 'imagine swimming between two panes of glass'). This approach (i.e., analogy learning) has been well received by our athletes with visual impairments, who have described the benefits of being able to visualise movements in their mind's eye. In addition, the coaching team is now exploring the use of analogies as a means of enhancing communication between coaches and athletes with intellectual impairments, where working memory capacity often hinders their ability to process more explicit instructions.

In assessing practice design, coaching sessions tended to comprise practice blocks which focused on a single skill for a large period of time. These blocks often took the form of part-task training, whereby skills are decomposed into component parts through the prescription of drills and then built progressively back into the full stroke or skill (e.g., the full swimming stroke is first reduced to the kick component, before adding in the arms and breathing). This technique is common in swimming training (see also Brackley et al., 2020), but the extent to which it facilitates the transfer of skills to other performance contexts remains an area of debate within SA literature and is perhaps indicative of the disconnect between theory and practice (Barris et al., 2013; Seifert et al., 2013). This notwithstanding, it was apparent that progression through isolated part-task drills or blocks comprising high volumes of repetition (as opposed to any process of switching *back and forth*) provided little opportunity to explore learning or different levels of challenge for the athlete.

Through discussions with the coaches regarding the potential impact of increased variability, the programme began experimenting with the scheduling of practice trials. Coaches would provide their plans for the session, and without changing the prescribed volume (typically the priority), the SA specialist highlighted ways to break large practice blocks down into smaller ones and distribute them across the session. For example, rather than practicing ten dives at the end of a session, a swimmer might practice three at the start, four in the middle, and three at the end. Within-skill variations could also be incorporated where necessary to promote movement exploration. It was reinforced to coaches that, although learning may not be immediately observable and may even be characterised by increased errors in practice, the benefits could be explored and assessed in 'race sets' at the end of the week designed to more closely replicate the performance context. Importantly, variability in practice was something the swimmers enjoyed!

Although coaches were using predominantly more prescriptive techniques such as part-task training, observations suggested there may have been attempts to align some task designs more closely with contemporary nonlinear approaches. However, it was clear that these were not under-pinned by an understanding of key concepts of the approach, such as self-organisation under constraints. As an example, one of the coaches removed the wall during turn practice (which could be considered a task constraint, see Newell & Jordan, 2007) to encourage their swimmer to get into the kick phase faster without the aid of the wall to gain propulsion. Interviews with coaches revealed that such techniques aimed to further enhance explicit (declarative) cognitive processes such as athlete awareness and under-standing of movements, in contrast with research recommendations that constraints should be designed and associated with more implicit (non-declarative) learning pathways (Brocken et al., 2020). This blurred line between explicit and implicit learning manifested in coaches adopting prescriptive instruction and feedback methods alongside the use of con-straints during practice (e.g., 'the principle of this drill is I'm trying to get you to kick your legs straight away when you've turned' – Powell et al., 2021, p. 1106). Furthermore, the coaches felt that regardless of how a skill is learned (with or without explicit skill knowledge) it should be demon-strated through verbal feedback and reflection from the swimmer (e.g., 'so we'll try and make a difference but could he actually feel there had been any difference and then feedback for myself on why they were observed as well' – Powell et al., 2021, p. 1106). Based on these insights, part of the current focus with BPS involves experimenting with the role of constraints as a means of replacing or reducing reliance on explicit instruction and allowing the athlete to explore the movement more freely before reflection and dialogue with the coach.

II. Empirical and applied interventions

Case study one neatly highlights the importance of researchers and prac-titioners immersing themselves in the context, and understanding 'where the coach is' (e.g., current knowledge, rationale for design, socio-cultural barriers), the gaps between research and coaching practice, and therefore, how to begin to address how to design better learning environments. Empirical approaches are vital to continue to improve our knowledge of Para sport contexts, which must move beyond snapshots of coaching be-haviours, and to promote collaborations between coaches and SA practi-tioners. As highlighted above, very few learning interventions in elite Para sport have been reported in the literature. One exception is Oudejans et al. (2012), where findings from basketball were creatively adapted and ex-plored in wheelchair basketball to improve information use during shooting. Importantly, the research highlighted that the principles of visual control in basketball shooting are similar between non-disabled and wheelchair disciplines. Given also that most Para sport coaches have developed in non-disabled sport pathways (Cregan et al., 2007), more research is needed to better explore how existing ideas and concepts from different contexts can be translated to Para sport contexts, and researchers and practitioners need to continue to look for ways to explore and embrace complex designs to cater for athletes with impairments.

Para sport contexts provide rich opportunities for innovative approaches for coach and athlete development (Askew et al., 2021) and could be used to epitomise the use of constraint-led approaches (CLA) to learning while considering the variation across impairment-related factors. Like Case study one (also see Powell et al., 2021), our work in an Australian context demonstrates the potential impact of applied SA supporting this process. Described in detail elsewhere, the lead author (Pinder) demonstrated how the use of design thinking and CLA in collaboration with a coach supported the technical development of a Paralympic long jumper (Pinder & Renshaw, 2019). To optimise learning and transfer to competition, constraints need to be used in a principled and systematic way. Building on concepts discussed above, simplified tasks representative of competition formats (rather than decomposed or part-task designs typical in long-jump training) were designed in a safe indoor environment in collaboration with the coach and athlete. This intervention resulted in technical changes that transferred to the outdoor environment.

This next level of 'embedding' SA specialists within multidisciplinary teams in Paralympic programs allows them to act as a mentor and facilitator of empirical and theoretical research and have greater scope to influence change; this has been shown to provide individualised support for both coach and athlete learning *in context* (Griffiths et al., 2018, Pinder et al., 2020). As a result, specialists embedded within elite programs afford coaches and athletes the opportunity to: (i) be consistently challenged, (ii) reflect on their current practices based on existing and emerging research evidence, and iii) co-create even better learning environments. We have shown that this ongoing and iterative approach (i.e., 'scaffolding' of knowledge and evolving practice), underpinned by key skills of SA specialists (e.g., logical presentation of ideas based on socio-cultural context, ability to engage athletes and build trust) can result in shifts in coaching philosophy and learning designs across both Paralympic and Olympic programs (Dehghansai et al., 2020a).

III. SA specialists supporting co-creation of the DPE

Taking a nonlinear approach to development emphasises the interaction between the individual and the environment, which is seen as central to optimising development (Ribeiro et al., 2021). We have also already recognised above that context is equally as important for coach learning as it is for athlete learning. Just as athletes learn to adapt and execute skills while guided by their coach, coaches themselves need the opportunity to explore (and sometimes fail) in order to further develop their ability to design effective learning environments. Coaches have recently been conceptualised as learning designers (Woods et al., 2020) and in Para sport in Australia they collaborate with SA specialists as part of a coach-athlete-practitioner relationship to find individual athlete performance solutions. This is significantly different to the traditional view of coaching – one where the coach directs the athlete through pre-determined and linear progressions via the provision of typically high volumes of instruction (Davids, 2015). Instead, co-created training session design places the athlete's development needs at the core of the coaching process. It draws upon the invaluable knowledge of lived experience of the athlete and utilises immersed support from mentors such as SA specialists to individualise and optimise training. Co-creation is practical to optimise Paralympic contexts, which by the inherent complex nature already requires coaches to be highly adaptable when designing and delivering training sessions that cater to individual athlete's developmental needs. We explore another example of how this can work in Case study two.

Case study II – Supporting co-creation and learning in Australian Para Athletics

Introduction and context

This case study presents an example of a SA specialist supporting co-creation of the DPE with a coach and two athletes (Para Javelin). The initiation of support involved an important (approximate) six-week period of integration in training, in addition to multiple one-on-one informal reflective discussions with the coach. This period enabled the SA specialist to build empathy and relationships with the coach and athletes – exploring and understanding their personalities, abilities, insights, and learning goals/needs. This also provided opportunity to observe key aspects of the environment that could be leveraged to support co-creation and learning (e.g., task design and progressions, coach-athlete interactions). As a former thrower and Paralympian, the coach's invaluable experiential knowledge of Para Throws events was harnessed (Greenwood et al., 2014), along with two critical components of their coaching philosophy. First, they viewed their relationship with their athletes as a 'performance partnership', emphasising a collaborative and individual athlete focus. Second, they proactively encouraged a 'check and challenge' environment where questions (from the athletes and support staff) were seen as constructive opportunities to (re-)evaluate and learn. Leveraging these experiential and philosophical aspects enabled a productive relationship to be formed between the SA specialist and the coach and, in turn, the athletes and underpinned the successful co-designed evolution of the DTE and the learnings for all parties.

Part 1 – Task design

Coach-athlete interactions appeared to occur spontaneously throughout a session and were typically aligned with exploring athlete's self-perception of technical positions, however, they were more commonly initiated by the coach and occasionally were focused on simply cross-checking drill purpose (for example, coach asking, *'what is the purpose of this drill?'* or, *'what does this drill target?'*). Further, static drills (i.e., stationary, non-throwing) were explained to be used to reinforce 'feel' of desirable technical positions and allowed the athletes to 'get into' those positions with a high degree of success (the reader may note the similarities in Para Swimming coaches' use of technical drills and cues from Case study one).

These insights provided a rich opportunity to support the coach in structuring more learning opportunities for their athletes, which challenged and refined their (already progressive) coaching philosophy. First, the SA specialist supported a shift in the coach and athletes' thinking regarding the design and structure of training tasks. Embracing the 'check and challenge' opportunity, the SA specialist facilitated group discussion which questioned the role of decomposed (part-task) and static drills for supporting the development of an inherently explosive and dynamic skill. It was collectively agreed that there was opportunity to enhance the design of drills by evolving them into more 'dynamic' iterations. These tasks encouraged athletes to explore moving 'through' (i.e., into and out of) various technical positions, at different speeds, while holding different weights or implements. Athlete-led feedback and insights focused on 'feel' were encouraged, however, discussion expanded to exploring athlete self-perceptions of differences or changes in 'feel' (as opposed to trying to find a specific feeling). Links to broader outcomes (e.g., actually throwing a ball or stick into a hanging net) were also included.

Part 2 – Session design

A second opportunity for co-design related to the overall sequence of tasks completed throughout a session. The coach and athletes were challenged to reflect on the blocked nature of completing all drills ahead of a single set of full throws, and whether this sequence facilitated or constrained available opportunities to develop constructive insights and transfer skills/ learning (i.e., from isolated, static technical positions directly to full techniques, which included performance outcomes – Merbah & Meulmans, 2011). The coach explores alternate session structures to test athlete insights, or 'check for transfer'. This involved more purposeful full throws (typically completed as smaller sets than previously described) interspersed around periods of dynamic tasks (e.g., varied drills). Drills were used to stimulate discussion and enabled each athlete to identify a key technical aspect, 'feeling' or idea that they wanted to transfer into a set of full throws (before returning to drills and repeating the unstructured, explorative drill-full throw cycle). The SA specialist supported the coach in evolving an environment to one which placed a greater emphasis on encouraging each athlete to find an individual solution to the challenge of 'learning to throw', as opposed to one that valued and prioritised athletes being able to feel and consistently execute 'correct' technical positions in static drills.

Part 3 – Exploring functional variability

Through these design shifts and collaborative discussions, the concept of an individualised technical 'bandwidth' emerged, which highlighted the importance of supporting each athlete to understand what technical 'range' (as opposed to a singular model) was critical to enabling them to sustain successful performance. Conceptually, this discussion was grounded on the notion of functional movement variability, a marker of performance previously thought to represent inconsistent (or 'poor') technical execution of skills or performance outcomes, now more commonly recognised as a defining characteristic of sport expertise (Seifert et al., 2013; Orth et al., 2017). In practice, this discussion shifted the collective thinking from 'feeling' (and executing) specific positions to establishing what was technically functional for each athlete and what opportunities (for technique development) could be exploited within the boundaries of the event rules. For example, time was spent exploring how (much of) the *full* dimensions of the runway could be optimally used in the run-up to facilitate successful technical execution and understanding how this impacted throw distance. This exploration enabled collaborative learning that some technical components had relatively more (e.g., angles and direction of movement during the run-up) and less (e.g., orientation of the front foot in the throwing position) functional variability (i.e., 'range') before performance decrement was observed, and were specific to the athlete. From a theoretical perspective this learning provides some indication of movement *degeneracy*, where different ranges of structural (i.e., technical) components can be utilised to achieve similar outcomes (i.e., performance outcomes, such as throw distance – Seifert et al., 2016). Finally, the coach reflected that the concept of exploring 'bandwidth' helped to highlight the importance of 'execution without perfection'.

The shifts in thinking briefly outlined here for training task and session designs created further opportunity to evolve these aspects to include short (periodised) cycles which incorporated a greater focus on 'performing' (Farrow & Robertson, 2017). During reflective discussions, the athletes highlighted that mixing exploration with performance sessions would enhance their own understanding of transfer between practicing the fundamental throwing skills and overall throwing performance. Consequently, a two-week learning cycle of six sessions was co-designed, which involved two cycles through a session focus structure of 'explore-transfer-perform'. The 'explore' component was underpinned by a compilation of notes and ideas developed collaboratively by the athlete, coach and SA specialist while the 'perform' sessions involved refined measures, such as capturing performance outcomes (i.e., throw distance), in 'bandwidth' blocks (Figure 8.2). Further, the athletes aimed to carry a limited number of concepts (1–2) through the cycle. This evolution of co-designing purposefully structured sessions with specific overall objectives emerged and was refined over an approximate six-month period, enhanced the variety of the DPE for the athletes, and supported deeper collective insight and understanding of learning and performance.

Summary

Case study two provided further insights into the practical application of SA theory and principles from a specialist embedded within the DPE. The examples provided highlighted the importance of coach-athlete-practitioner relationship (see Dehghansai et al., 2020b) and suggested that big shifts in thinking can occur over a relatively short period of time. The strategic use of SA specialists to support co-creation of coach and athlete development in Para sport contexts can not only have significant impacts on learning design but could help reduce some of the challenges associated with high-performance Para sport environments (e.g., limited resources or experienced coaches, limited development opportunities). Future work should focus on developing innovative research programs to better capture coach and athlete challenges and explore the role of SA specialists across athlete and coach talent pathways.

Practitioner commentary

Over the past decades sport sciences and human movement sciences have gathered much information on talent development and skill acquisition in sports. The challenge we are now facing is how we bring all this knowledge, that was gathered mainly in relatively 'fundamental' studies, to actual practice, that is, to coaches, athletes and sporting organizations who work on a daily basis on the development of their skills. This is the case for non-disabled sport as much as for Para sports. The challenge is even bigger than

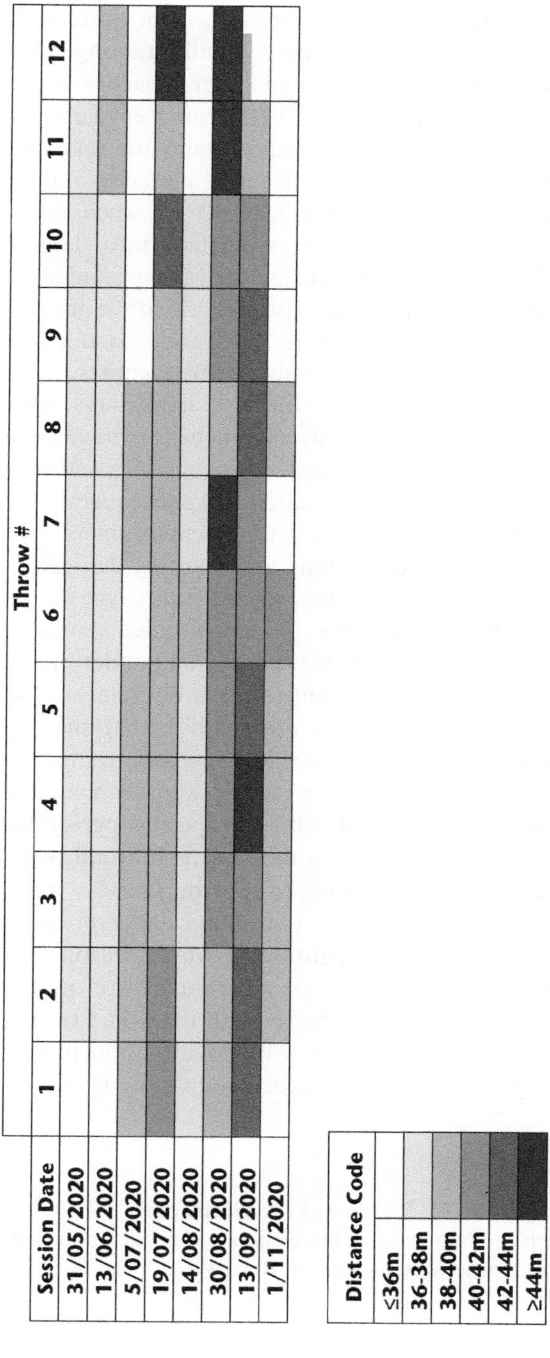

FIGURE 8.2 An example of monitoring 'bandwidth' performance outcomes

you might think because just knowing a great deal about evidence-based practice methods (i.e., methods of which we know they have much potential to speed up the development of expertise) is far from sufficient to be able to actually use this knowledge appropriately in daily training environments. It is a complex process that involves stakeholder (coaches, athletes, organizations) buy-in as well as co-creation of learning environments: two elements we have only recently started to understand and take into account in our efforts to develop evidence-based training methods in daily practice.

This is eloquently described in this Chapter. As such, the approach of embedding skill acquisition or other specialists into daily training environments is definitely an important step forward, provided that sufficient resources are available of course; the cases described are great examples but definitely not resource free. Therefore, it is good to think of structural cooperation between researchers, (embedded) scientists, sport organizations, coaches, and athletes in the form of living labs where scientists support coaches and athletes in the development of evidence-based training methods. More importantly, this needs to occur in a setting where these methods can immediately be implemented and subsequently evaluated; not in a lab at the university but in the natural environment of the athletes, ensuring representativeness of training and learning designs.

Undoubtedly, Para sports has its own challenges, yet the processes and cases described in this Chapter apply to non-disabled sports as much as to Para sports. One important example is performing under pressure, which is not something restricted to non-disabled sports but relevant for Para sport, as well as any other performance domain for that matter. Using the constraints-led approach to (co-)design learning and training environments that at some point and to a certain degree approach and represent the actual performance environment with its specific performance circumstances (such as high pressure) is equally valuable to all performance domains and environments. When and for how long certain training methods (e.g., frequency and volume), such as training under pressure, should be done preparing for specific competition, a whole season, a whole talent development program with a team or individually are questions we have only recently started to unravel, exactly with cases like those described in the Chapter. More work like these will provide opportunities to further develop and apply skill acquisition expertise in daily training practice.

References

Askew, G. A., Pinder, R. A., Renshaw, I., & Gorman, A. (2021). Elite coaching in Para-sport: Rich environments for innovation in coach development. *International Journal of Sport Science & Coaching*. In Review.

Barris, S., Davids, K., & Farrow, D. (2013). Representative learning design in springboard diving: Is dry-land training representative of a pool dive?. *European Journal of Sport Science, 13*(6), 638–645.

Brackley, V., Barris, S., Tor, E., & Farrow, D. (2020). Coaches' perspective towards skill acquisition in swimming: What practice approaches are typically applied in training? *Journal of Sports Sciences, 38*(22), 2532–2542.

Brocken, J. E. A., van der Kamp, J., Lenoir, M., & Savelsbergh, G. J. P. (2020). Equipment modification can enhance skill learning in young field hockey players. *International Journal of Sports Science & Coaching, 15*(3), 382–389.

Cregan, K., Bloom, G. A., & Reid, G. (2007). Career evolution and knowledge of elite coaches of swimmers with a physical disability. *Research Quarterly for Exercise and Sport, 78*(4), 339–350.

Davids, K. (2015). Athletes and sports teams as complex adaptive system: A review of implications for learning design. *Revista Internacional De Ciencias Del Deporte, 11*(39), 48–61.

Dehghansai, N., Headrick, J., Renshaw, I., Pinder, R. A., & Barris, S. (2020a). Olympic and Paralympic coach perspectives on effective skill acquisition support and coach development. *Sport, Education and Society, 25*(6), 667–680.

Dehghansai, N., Lemez, S., Wattie, N., & Baker, J. (2017). A systematic review of influences on development of athletes with disabilities. *Adapted Physical Activity Quarterly, 34*(1), 72–90.

Dehghansai, N., Lemez, S., Wattie, N., Pinder, R. A., & Baker, J. (2020b). Understanding the development of elite parasport athletes using a constraint-led approach: Considerations for coaches and practitioners. *Frontiers in Psychology, 11*, 2612.

Fairhurst, K. E., Bloom, G. A., & Harvey, W. J. (2017). The learning and mentoring experiences of Paralympic coaches. *Disability and Health Journal, 10*(2), 240–246.

Farrow, D., & Robertson, S. (2017). Development of a skill acquisition periodisation framework for high-performance sport. *Sports Medicine, 47*(6), 1043–1054.

Greenwood, D., Davids, K., & Renshaw, I. (2014). Experiential knowledge of expert coaches can help identify informational constraints on performance of dynamics interceptive actions. *Journal of Sports Sciences, 32*(4), 328–335.

Griffiths, M. A., Armour, K. M., & Cushion, C. J. (2018). 'Trying to get our message across': Successes and challenges in an evidence-based professional development programme for sport coaches. *Sport, Education and Society, 23*(3), 283–295.

Kearney, P. E., Carson, H. J., & Collins, D., (2018). Implementing technical refinement in high-level athletics: Exploring the knowledge schemas of coaches. *Journal of Sports Sciences, 36*(10), 1118–1126.

Masters, R. S., van Duijn, T., & Uiga, L. (2019). Advances in implicit motor learning. In Masters, R. S. & Poolton, J. M. (Eds.), *Skill acquisition in Sport* (pp. 77–96). Routledge.

McMaster, S., Culver, D., & Werthner, P. (2012). Coaches of athletes with a physical disability: A look at their learning experiences. *Qualitative Research in Sport, Exercise and Health, 4*(2), 226–243.

Merbah, S., & Meulmans, T. (2011). Learning a motor skill: Effects of blocked versus random practice – A review. *Psychologica Belgica, 51*(1), 15–48.

Moy, B., Renshaw, I., Davids, K., & Brymer, E. (2016). Overcoming acculturation: Physical education recruits' experiences of an alternative pedagogical approach to games teaching. *Physical Education and Sport Pedagogy, 21*(4), 386–406.

Mullen, R., Faull, A., Jones, E. S., & Kingston, K. (2015). Evidence for the effectiveness of holistic process goals for learning and performance under pressure. *Psychology of Sport and Exercise, 17*, 40–44.

Newell, K. M., & Jordan, K. (2007). Task constraints and movement organization: A common language. In Davis, W. E. & Broadhead, G. D. (Eds.), *Ecological task analysis and movement* (pp. 5–23). Champaign, IL: Human Kinetics.

Orth, D., Van der Kamp, J., Memmert, D., & Savelsbergh, G. J. (2017). Creative motor actions as emerging from movement variability. *Frontiers in Psychology, 8*, 1903.

Oudejans, R. R., Heubers, S., Ruitenbeek, J. R. J., & Janssen, T. W. (2012). Training visual control in wheelchair basketball shooting. *Research Quarterly for Exercise and Sport, 83*(3), 464–469.

Paulson, T., & Goosey-Tolfrey, V. (2017). Current perspectives on profiling and enhancing wheelchair court sport performance. *International Journal of Sports Physiology and Performance, 12*(3), 275–286.

Pinder, R. A., Maloney, M., Renshaw, I., & Barris, S. (2020). The role of skill acquisition specialists in talent development. In *Talent identification and development in Sport* (pp. 130–144). Routledge.

Pinder, R. A., & Renshaw, I. (2019). What can coaches and physical education teachers learn from a constraints-led approach in para-sport? *Physical Education and Sport Pedagogy, 24*(2), 190–205.

Powell, D., Wood, G., Kearney, P. E., & Payton, C. (2021). Skill acquisition practices of coaches on the British Para swimming World Class Programme. *International Journal of Sports Science & Coaching, 16*(5) 1097–1110.

Ribeiro, J., Davids, K., Silva, P., Coutinho, P., Barreira, D., & Garganta, J. (2021). Talent development in sport requires athlete enrichment: Contemporary insights from a nonlinear pedagogy and the athletic skills model. *Sports Medicine, 51*(6), 1115–1122.

Seifert, L., Button, C., & Davids, K. (2013). Key properties of expert movement systems in sport. *Sports medicine, 43*(3), 167–178.

Seifert, L., Komar, J., Araújo, D., & Davids, K. (2016). Neurobiological degeneracy: A key property for functional adaptations of perception and action to constraints. *Neuroscience & Behavioral Reviews, 69*, 159–165.

Stodter, A., & Cushion, C. J. (2019). Evidencing the impact of coaches' learning: Changes in coaching knowledge and practice over time. *Journal of Sports Sciences, 37*(18), 2086–2093.

Townsend, R. C., Huntley, T. D., Cushion, C. J., & Culver, D. (2021). Infusing disability into coach education and development: A critical review and agenda for change. *Physical Education and Sport Pedagogy*. Advance online publication.

Woods, C. T., McKeown, I., Rothwell, M., Araújo, D., Robertson, S., & Davids, K. (2020). Sport practitioners as sport ecology designers: How ecological dynamics has progressively changed perceptions of skill "acquisition" in the sporting habitat. *Frontiers in Psychology, 11*(654), 1–15.

Wulf, G. (2013). Attentional focus and motor learning: A review of 15 years. *International Review of Sport and Exercise Psychology, 6*(1), 77–104.

9

TALENT TRANSFER IN PARALYMPIC SPORT

Nima Dehghansai and Adeline Green
Practitioner Commentary: Melissa Wilson

Introduction

The increase in quality and depth of international competition has seen sporting organizations[1] around the world develop new and innovative talent identification and development strategies with the goal of continued success at the highest level. A recent initiative that has gained interest within athlete development settings is talent transfer, which typically refers to an accelerated talent development pathway where an athlete who has reached an elite level in one sport (the 'donor sport'), transitions to a new sport (the 'recipient sport') with the goal of achieving elite-level success (Collins et al., 2014; MacNamara & Collins, 2015; Rea & Lavallee, 2015, 2017).

Talent transfer in Paralympic contexts

In no other sport contexts are there as many examples of talent transfer as in Paralympic sport. There are numerous examples of athletes who have been able to reach the elite level in multiple sports, occasionally in both Summer and Winter sports, and sometimes even simultaneously! Early in the Paralympic Games history (see Chapter 2), it was not uncommon for athletes to compete in multiple sports at the one Games. This can probably be attributed to low Paralympic sport participation rates, and therefore small teams for each country, in addition to lack of funding for athletes and teams to travel internationally to a Games. Therefore, it was highly likely that even though an athlete's main sport might have been, for example, Para swimming, the athlete may have been called upon to make up the numbers in a team sport, such as Wheelchair Basketball, just so the team could compete.

DOI: 10.4324/9781003184430-9

As Paralympic sports have become more competitive over time, due to the increase in participation rates and talent pools as well as an increase in high-performance support, multi-sport and talent transfer athletes have become less common. That said, there are well-known examples of athletes who have been able to excel in multiple sports. Using Australia at the Tokyo 2020 Paralympic Games as an example, the Paralympic team had at least five athletes who had competed in another sport at a different Games including: Daniela di Toro (Wheelchair Tennis/Para Table Tennis), Michael Auprince (Para Swimming/Wheelchair Basketball), Dylan Alcott (Wheelchair Basketball/Wheelchair Tennis), Amanda Reid (Para Swimming/Para Cycling), and Hannah Dodd (Para Equestrian/Wheelchair Basketball). More broadly, since the first Paralympic Games in 1960, over one hundred Australian Paralympians have competed in two or more Paralympic sports with Dylan Alcott becoming one of the most recent Australian Paralympians to win Gold medals in two different sports (Wheelchair Basketball in 2008 and Wheelchair Tennis in 2016 and 2020). There are even instances of athletes being able to transfer their skills and attributes between Winter and Summer Paralympic sports simultaneously, such as Jessica Gallagher, who represented Australia in three different sports (Para Alpine skiing, Para Athletics, and Para Cycling) across four different Winter and Summer Paralympic Games (Vancouver 2010, London 2012, Sochi 2014, Rio 2016), winning three bronze medals in three of the Games with two different sports. While significantly less common, there are also athletes who have competed dually both in the Olympic and Paralympic Games, usually in the same sport (e.g., Melissa Tapper, Table Tennis and Para Table Tennis).

In this chapter, we unpack the process of transfer and explore the limited literature to better understand what we currently know of the transfer process. First, we present some previous and current talent transfer programs and initiatives[2] in non-disabled and Para contexts. At the same time, the various transfer opportunities along the pathway will be discussed. We then explore the array of reasons athletes consider a transfer, along with the underlying benefits for the athletes and factors that contribute to sport organizations' decisions to embed transfer into their pathway systems. We conclude the chapter by examining Para-specific challenges to transfer and provide a list of considerations that can contribute to an optimal transfer process.

Embedding transfer into sporting pathways

Talent transfer is based upon the notion that athletes can maximize investments made in a 'donor sport' by transferring aspects of their acquired expertise and accelerating development in their new sport. The time taken for a talent transfer athlete to achieve an elite level in the new sport is, therefore, expected to be quicker than the typical route through the development pathway in the 'recipient sport'. Thus, talent transfer may increase the chance of identifying athletes who can attain international success by reducing talent development timeframes and thereby increasing return on investment in athlete development (Vaeyens et al., 2009).

Current practices in non-disabled contexts

Sports that implement talent transfer programs to attract new talent often explicitly aim to target athletes from sports with similar characteristics. An example of this is Project Phoenix, a national partnership between the Australian Institute of Sport, Gymnastics Australia, the Olympic Winter Institute of Australia, and Diving Australia. Project Phoenix provides gymnasts with the opportunity to transfer their athletic ability to a new sport such as Diving, Aerial Skiing, Pole-Vault or Sport Climbing (Gymnastics Australia, n.d.). Based on these similar physiological, anthropometric and skill characteristics athletes are expected to develop more rapidly since they utilize previously learned skills or attributes to maximize learning and development in their new sport (Bullock et al., 2009). Other sport organizations have taken similar approaches targeting experienced athletes with specific anthropometric or physiological characteristics. Examples of such talent transfer programs include the U.K. Sport 'Tall and Talented' and 'Sporting Giants', which aimed to recruit 'taller' athletes with sporting backgrounds into Rowing, Handball, and Volleyball, claiming these traits to be advantageous (UK Sport, 2010, 2012). This is supported by research highlighting the possibility of successful transfer between sports with similar characteristics (i.e., sprinting and skeleton both require power; ball team sports require similar tactical skills, running and cross-country skiing both require athletes with high aerobic capacity, etc., Bullock et al., 2009). However, qualitative studies investigating the perspectives of athletes, coaches, and performance support staff on talent transfer have argued the similarities between sports does not fully account for successful talent transfer (Collins et al., 2014; Rea & Lavallee, 2015, 2017) and there is uncertainty regarding whether this similarity is sufficient for a successful transfer within Para contexts (Dehghansai & Baker, 2022; Dehghansai et al., 2022).

Para sport transfer programs

Internationally, talent transfer programs are being integrated into sport pathways and recruitment programs in Paralympic sport (see Chapter 4), as sport organisations search for new strategies to increase the pool of athletes, with the ultimate goal of increased success at the elite level. One of the goals of the Canadian Paralympic Committee's *Paralympian Search,* for example, is to identify opportunities for athletes looking to transfer between sports (Dehghansai & Baker, 2020). While in non-disabled contexts, discussions of talent transfer occur mostly within high-performance settings, programs in Para contexts also focus on lesser-skilled athletes already in a pathway, or those with acquired impairments who may not have experience in Para sport (but come with experience in non-disabled contexts). There are programs like Paralympian Search that are very structured, where the leading organization (e.g., Canadian Paralympic Committee) facilitates the sessions, coordinates testing stations and capturing of data, and welcomes sports to engage with athletes during the events.

Similarly, another group who may find Para sport transfer opportunities are military personnel injured during active service. Whilst this may not fit existing talent transfer definitions (i.e., elite sport to sport), veterans often have extensive training histories in addition to many beneficial psychological characteristics (e.g., motivation and resilience) that have been described as essential for talent transfer (MacNamara & Collins, 2015). There are specific programs (e.g., Canada's Soldier On program) that are tied to the Invictus Games, a biannual competition designed specifically to provide opportunities for injured veterans looking to get into Para sports. Other initiatives are less structured and can involve collaborations between different sports with similar demands (e.g., Para Swimming, Para Cycling, Para Rowing) or sport-specific initiatives designed for athletes to 'come and try' the activity. Other initiatives which mainly focus on entry point transfers involve collaborations with schools and rehabilitation programs. Collectively, the common goal of these programs and initiatives is to provide opportunities for persons with impairments to sample sports and become aware of opportunities that exist within their communities. This, ultimately, will increase the pool of athletes in the system while providing the select few the opportunity to embark on the high-performance journey.

Benefits and challenges of talent transfer

Talent transfer programs are currently utilized by numerous sporting organizations, institutes, and academies around the world with the principle aim of maximizing sport success. Many benefits and advantages of talent transfer have been proposed for both the athlete and the sport organisation, with intentions and experiences varying for each stakeholder.

Benefits for the athlete

Athletes competing in high-performance settings tend to develop strong athletic identities throughout their careers and thus, retirement can be a very difficult phase for athletes to cope with (Grove et al., 1996). This is exacerbated when athletes are faced with a nonnormative career-changing experience (e.g., career-ending injury, changes in classification system deeming them ineligible in their current sport; Van de Vliet et al., 2008). One argument for a talent transfer pathway is that it provides athletes with a 'second chance' (Dehghansai & Baker, 2021; MacNamara & Collins, 2015). An athlete may consider leaving their donor sport for various reasons, including age (especially in sports with the relatively young age of peak performance), deselection from a team, plateaus in development, burnout, or career-ending injuries (Dehghansai & Baker, 2021). Some may also leave their donor sport if they feel they have accomplished all they can in that sport, from either exceeding their own expectations and goals, or due to a lack of a sport pathway to higher levels of competition (e.g., international level) (Dehghansai & Baker, 2021). When an athlete feels they have skills and capacities that can be applied to a new sport, talent transfer can provide an opportunity for them to extend their career and time at the elite level (Gulbin & Ackland, 2008; Vaeyens et al., 2009). Therefore, athletes can use talent transfer to enjoy the physical, psychological, and social benefits associated with sport or move into new challenges.

There are also elements unique to Paralympic sport athletes' experiences, mainly due to nonnormative events. For example, occasionally athletes in Paralympic sports may undergo a classification review that results in (re) classification or with them being deemed ineligible. This can be due to impairment-related changes for the athlete (e.g., due to a degenerative condition) or classification rule alterations by the sport governing body. A change in classification can result in the athlete competing in classes where they are less competitive (either due to impairment-related reasons or depth of the class pool) and therefore have a reduced probability of success. An athlete in this situation may consider transfer as an option to continue training with the potential to compete at an international level. Relatedly, athletes are sometimes unable to continue to compete in their original sport if they experience changes in their impairment due to a progressive disease which may result in the removal or revision of their classification status in their sport (see more on classification-related outcomes in Chapter 6). Transfer opportunities allow the athlete to explore opportunities in another sport. Sport-specific injuries could also be a reason for exploring transfer such as when a Para athlete explores other Para sports (e.g., the transition from Wheelchair Tennis to Para Table Tennis post-injury) or when an athlete with a newly acquired impairment transfers from non-disabled sports to Para sports (e.g., Basketball to Wheelchair Basketball, given their impairment is eligible for classification). Thus, providing athletes with alternatives to retirement that keep them in sport and prolong their careers can reduce the negative effects (e.g., lower self-esteem or loss of identity) associated with involuntary retirement while continuing to provide the physical, psychological, and social benefits associated with sport participation (Marin-Urquiza et al., 2018).

Benefits for the sport organisation

At the organisational level, talent transfer may increase success in sports where a talent 'gap' exists. A talent transfer pathway can provide fast-tracked development that increases the chance of international success for sports that are not currently competitive or have a smaller talent pool (Bullock et al., 2009). For example, Para Badminton, recently included at the Paralympic Games, may benefit from welcoming high-performance athletes from Wheelchair Tennis with extensive experience at the international stage. Not only these athletes may be able to transfer their skills into the new sport and fast track to compete at the high-performance stage sooner, but they can also act as mentors for novice athletes just entering the Para Badminton system. In addition, well-established sports could also benefit from an athlete transfer, if they identify a gap in a specific discipline. For example, Para Cycling may identify a specific discipline that internationally has a small pool of competitors and support a transfer athlete from Para Athletics to develop sport-specific skills to advance their careers in that Para Cycling discipline. Considering the athlete may have already been exposed to high-performance training, this allows Para Cycling to focus more on the sport-specific skills and devote less time to developing the fundamental high-performance skills that the athlete had exposure to (i.e., self-regulation techniques, nutrition knowledge, etc.).

Sport organizations invest significant resources into talent identification and development programs that generally have low or inconsistent success rates (Baker et al., 2018). Talent transfer can reduce the range of resources needed to develop the athlete due to their pre-existing skills (developed visuomotor capacities, a more robust physiological, physical, and psychological readiness) and knowledge associated with the high-performance sport (i.e., awareness of nutritional guidelines, training periodization). Furthermore, by targeting athletes who have knowledge and experience of the high-performance sport system and what is required (training volume, psychological characteristics) to achieve success, the accuracy rate of talent identification and development programs may be improved (Dehghansai & Baker, 2021; Vaeyens et al., 2009). However, it is important for sports to have a clear understanding of gaps within their system, both domestically and internationally, in order to provide appropriate opportunities for athletes that fit those profiles. As a result, talent transfer may have even greater implications for Para sport organizations where athlete retention is critical for athlete development and the overall health and efficiency of the

Paralympic system. Thus, if implemented effectively, talent transfer can increase both athlete retention and Paralympic success.

Challenges with Para sport transfer

Within Para sport, research investigating factors that act as a facilitator or barrier for either formal or informal talent transfers is scarce (Dehghansai & Baker, 2021). Whilst there are sure to be commonalities between non-disabled and Para sport talent transfer, other factors are likely to be substantially different. For example, Paralympic sport has unique characteristics pertaining to impairment-related factors including classification (see Chapter 6) and specialized equipment (see Chapter 11). Paralympic athletes also face distinct challenges and barriers when striving for sporting success, such as issues with accessing training facilities and high-quality coaches with Para sport experiences (see Chapter 7 on quality experience to increase retention in Paralympic sport). These contextual factors should be considered by practitioners working with transfer athletes in Paralympic sport while Para-specific research is necessary to understand the interaction of these constraints on athletes' transfer experiences.

In a recent publication, Dehghansai et al. (2022) highlighted the tendency for athletes with acquired impairments to specialize in Paralympic sports that were similar to their non-disabled sports experiences. In addition, the only talent transfer work specific to Paralympic sport that we are aware of, done by Dehghansai and Baker (2022), not only highlighted the importance of considerations noted in the non-disabled literature (i.e., physical, psychological and environmental factors that impact transfer quality), but also accentuated key interpersonal factors and communication challenges associated with athletes' transfer. One of the key considerations emphasized was the importance of aligning expectations amongst all stakeholders (athlete, donor, and recipient sports), with an athlete-centered approach being the focus of any transfer process.

Considerations for talent transfer programs and initiatives

Based on the limited literature and current practices, there are number of factors that can contribute to a more successful talent transfer process. Below we highlight a few of these elements for consideration when designing and facilitating athlete transfer.

Athlete-centered focus

As noted earlier, ensuring that the program is designed considering the athlete's best interest at the forefront is a key component for ensuring beneficial transfer. This includes addressing some of the elements listed below including the type of resources available for the athletes during their adjustment period. It is also critical to understand the specific reasons why the athlete is exploring transfer opportunities and whether the recipient sport can fulfill these needs. Similarly, there may be differences between the training environments (e.g., daily training environment, sporting demands, teammate interactions, team versus individual sport setting), and how the new environment differentiates from their previous sport is vital to helping the athlete adjust to their new environments.

Provisional classification

As mentioned previously, existing talent transfer programs focus predominantly on physical characteristics and similarities between sports to ensure a successful transfer between sports (Collins et al., 2014; Rea & Lavallee, 2015, 2017). A significant consideration within the Paralympic sport contexts is athletes' provisional classification and the associated attributes (i.e., class depth, sporting demands for this specific sport class, etc.). Athletes' classification can impact their potential development in a specific sport. Whether the athlete is classified in a category that is favorable (e.g., are they classed at a higher or lower end of a specific class), and if that corresponding class has a competitive pool of athletes domestically or internationally can impact opportunities, resources, and ultimately, the rate at which the athlete can progress. Therefore, systemizing the process to ensure athlete classification occurs early in the transfer phase and having a dedicated staff to oversee this process is vital to aligning expectations and subsequent successful transfer outcomes.

Psychological attributes

Generally, athletes who have reached an elite level are known to be goal-oriented and outcome-focused with a strong athletic identity, and some athletes struggle with the loss of identity in their previous sport, contributing to the decision to seek a new environment (Dehghansai & Baker, 2021). However, changes in sporting demands (e.g., going from being an expert to a relative novice) can test athletes' resiliency and ability to cope with adversity (Collins et al., 2014; Dehghansai et al., 2021b). Therefore, athletes can benefit from psychological support during the acclimatisation period in their new sport.

Other psychological skills and characteristics including confidence, motivation, determination, commitment, mental strength, and self-belief are often overlooked during the talent transfer process (Collins et al., 2014; MacNamara & Collins, 2015). Unlike athletes entering a sport at a lower level of the pathway, talent transfer athletes may have already developed these qualities during their experience in their previous sports. Some researchers have argued that a shortcoming of talent transfer programs currently is that psychological factors are often overlooked and not operationalized in the initial phases of a formalized talent transfer program (Collins et al., 2014; MacNamara & Collins, 2015). The lack of representative design (see Pinder et al., 2011) and overreliance on physiological variables to inform decisions is another, related shortcoming within talent transfer initiatives (this is also a shortcoming in the recruitment space in Para sports, see Chapter 5).

Deliberate programming

While the list of resources for consideration here may seem elementary and important for success for any athlete entering a performance pathway, it is the unique elements related to an individual athlete's journey (i.e., the right things at the right time) that systematically need to be embedded in the transfer process during their transition period (Dehghansai & Baker, 2021). Provisional classification and psychological support are the primary components; however, it is equally important to ensure athletes have access to an expert coach who can develop individualized plans based on athlete's current circumstances (i.e., previous sporting experience, training history, injury record, impairment-related factors, etc.). Athletes may be accustomed to a specific style of training (e.g., consider sociocultural aspects of training in an individual sport versus team sport training environments) and physically, their training has exposed them to meet the demands of another sport. Thus, providing athletes with sufficient time to develop in the recipient sport, without pressure for strong performance outcomes early after the transfer, can be facilitative of a successful transfer while minimizing injuries and burnout (MacNamara & Collins, 2015). Accounting for these factors, amongst others, has been termed 'deliberate programming', referring to the strategic planning of any talent development program (not just with transfer) (Bullock et al., 2009). This may include providing access to a) expert coaches and other performance support staff, b) equipment, c) training camps and competition, and d) financial, technical, and medical support – all to ensure athletes have every opportunity to reach their full potential in the sport. For transfer athletes, the timing of their exposure to these resources can be vital for a successful acclimatization period.

Avoid a singular focus

Last, and most importantly, talent transfer should never be the only focus. Sport organizations should continue to develop talent through the entirety of the sport pathway in order to bring new athletes into the sport to ensure there are opportunities across the continuum and improve the overall health of the pathway. Talent transfer programs should be a part of the pathway, with structured guidelines and instructions to guide the transfer process, including communication, expectation, and resource allocation. Ultimately, this involves shifting away from talent transfer initiatives into talent transfer programs.

Concluding thoughts

There is limited research on talent transfer, especially in Para sport contexts. Therefore, our current understanding of the factors influencing successful talent transfer is limited and has generally been drawn from the non-disabled sport literature. Considering the nuances associated with athlete development in Para contexts, conclusions borrowed from the non-disabled literature should be done with caution. Nevertheless, this chapter has summarized some important considerations for athletes and stakeholders involved in the talent transfer programs, including a discussion of: the benefits of talent transfer for both athletes and stakeholders, the challenges that may be faced by athletes and sport organizations, the barriers and facilitators, and other specific factors that should be considered when involved with talent transfer in sport. Whilst talent transfer can never be the only talent identification and development pathway within a sport, it can provide exciting opportunities for athletes and sports organizations that support existing pathways and strategies.

Practitioner commentary

I couldn't agree more with the authors of this chapter, in that the opportunities for successful talent transfer are perhaps more evident and available in the Paralympic context than in any other sporting sphere. Not only have many Para athletes already demonstrated the possibilities of successful sport transfer, but as pointed out by the authors, the unique parameters of Para sport lend themselves perfectly to transfer opportunities. It is important for sport practitioners to be cognizant of these parameters (e.g., classification nuances, shorter developmental timeframes, acquired injuries, etc.) as drivers for the integration of talent transfer frameworks. Borrowing from my experience (both as a transfer athlete myself, and as a practitioner involved in transfers), I have provided some key takeaways for practitioners to consider:

1. Dedicated Para pathway personnel
    While resources are challenging in Para sport contexts, it is imperative that someone within the organisation has explicit responsibility for Para athlete development, who can coordinate talent transfer processes.

2. Evidenced-based athlete and event profiles

   A strong, holistic understanding of athlete success profiles specific to each event can a) help sports better understand the depth of the field, performance standards, competitor demographics, impairment profiles, and developmental trajectories of athletes, b) inform sports' decisions on how to approach transfer (and what to look for), and c) allow comparison of candidates' current capabilities against those required for success in the new sport.

3. Documented Para pathways

   All athletes should have a clear understanding of the progressive developmental stages from sport introduction to sport mastery (e.g., typical daily training environments, competition opportunities, support frameworks, performance benchmarks and athlete commitments) to help them understand and navigate the developmental environment (including transfer athletes just entering the system). While the general phases of athlete development are relatively standard across sports, there can be considerable variation in provisions and commitments between sports, so it is important for transfer athletes to be aware of these differences early to avoid confusion and manage expectations.

4. Specific talent transfer verification processes and support frameworks

   Despite displaying significant potential based on generic personal and physical attributes, transfer athletes may not qualify for funding or performance support via the traditional criteria due to a lack of sport-specific skills and competitive experience. As such, to enable transfer athletes to transition into their new sport rapidly, accommodations may be required to give athletes access to the support they need. While this may at times be perceived as unfair by traditional pathway athletes and stakeholders, in my experience, a clearly articulated 'sport transfer program' with specific support provisions and dedicated monitoring/verification processes can provide an appropriate and rationalised approach to eligibility and provision of support for transfer athletes.

5. Strong network relationships

   When Para pathway leads, coaches and/or support staff from different sporting organisations are well connected, intelligence regarding the athlete characteristics and impairment types associated with success for each sporting organisation become shared knowledge, and staff are in a better position to identify possible sport transfer opportunities, then initiate sport transfer conversations and processes when appropriate.

   It is important to note that the factors described above I deem to be beneficial but not *necessary* for successful talent transfer. As is the case for all aspects of athlete development, there is no 'secret formula' or 'one size fits all' approach, we can only share our experiences, learn from each other and explore what works for us within our own contexts.

Notes

1 Sport organization, unless stated otherwise, is used broadly to refer to national sport organizations, national governing bodies, national Paralympic committees and/or any stakeholder overseeing the infrastructure of a sport
2 In this chapter, program refers to an established structure with clear guidelines and instructions to attain a specific outcome, while initiative is preliminary inception of a plan to solve an existing problem.

References

Baker, J., Schorer, J., & Wattie, N. (2018). Compromising talent: Issues in identifying and selecting talent in sport. *Quest, 70*(1), 48–63.

Bullock, N., Gulbin, J. P., Martin, D. T., Ross, A., Holland, T., & Marino, F. (2009). Talent identification and deliberate programming in skeleton: Ice novice to Winter Olympian in 14 months. *Journal of Sports Sciences, 27*(4), 397–404.

Collins, R., Collins, D., MacNamara, A., & Jones, M. I. (2014). Change of plans: An evaluation of the effectiveness and underlying mechanisms of successful talent transfer. *Journal of Sports Sciences, 32*(17), 1621–1630.

Dehghansai, N. (2021). *A comprehensive analysis of the factors affecting the development of expertise in athletes with impairments* (Publication No. 38451) [Doctoral dissertation, York University]. York Space Institutional Repository.

Dehghansai, N., & Baker, J. (2022). (in review). Coach and athlete perspectives on talent transfer in Paralympic sport. *Adapted Physical Activity Quarterly*.

Dehghansai, N. & Baker, J. (2020). Searching for Paralympians: Characteristics of participants attending 'search' events. *Adapted Physical Activity Quarterly, 37*(1), 129–138.

Dehghansai, N., Pinder, R., & Baker, J. (2022). Pathways in Paralympic sport: An in-depth analysis of athletes' developmental trajectories and training histories. *Adapted Physical Activity Quarterly, 39*(1), 37–85.

Dehghansai, N., Pinder, R., & Baker, J. (2021b). "Looking for a golden needle in the haystack": Perspectives on talent identification and development in Paralympic sport. *Frontiers in Sports and Active Living: Elite Sports and Performance Enhancement, 3*, 635977.

Grove, J. R., Lavallee, D., & Gordon, S. (1996). Coping with retirement from sport: The influence of athletic identity. *Journal of Applied Sport Psychology, 9*(2), 191–203.

Gulbin, J. P., & Ackland, T. R., (2008). Talent identification and profiling. In T. R. Acklan, B. C. Elliott, & J. Bloomfield (Eds.), *Applied anatomy & biomechanics in sport* (2nd ed., pp. 60–72). Human Kinetics.

Gymnastics Australia. (n.d.). Gymnasts given increased sport pathway opportunities. Retrieved December 13, 2021 from https://www.gymnastics.org.au/Ga/Posts/News_Articles/2020/11_Nov/Gymnasts_given_increased_sport_pathway_opportunities.aspx

MacNamara, Á., & Collins, D. (2015). Second chances: Investigating athletes' experiences of talent transfer. *Plos One, 10*, 11.

Marin-Urquiza, A., Ferreira, J. P., & Van Biesen, D. (2018). Athletic identity and self-esteem among active and retired Paralympic athletes. *European Journal of Sport Science, 18*(6), 861–871.

Pinder, R. A., Davids, K., Renshaw, I., & Araújo, D. (2011). Representative learning design and functionality of research and practice in sport. *Journal of Sport Exercise and Psychology*, *33*(1), 146–155.

Rea, T., & Lavallee, D. (2015). An examination of athletes' experiences of the talent transfer process. *Talent Development & Excellence*, *7*(1), 41–67.

Rea, T., & Lavallee, D. (2017). The structured repsychling of talent. In J. Baker, S. Colbey, J. Schorer & N. Wattie, (Eds.), *Routledge handbook of talent identification and development in sport*. Routledge.

UK Sport. (2010). Tall and talented hopefuls face anxious wait. Retrieved December 13, 2021 from https://www.uksport.gov.uk/news/2010/02/11/tall-and-talented-hopefuls-face-anxious-wait

UK Sport. (2012). Sporting giants celebrate fifth anniversary. Retrieved December 13, 2021 from https://www.uksport.gov.uk/news/2012/02/27/sporting-giants-celebrate-fifth-anniversary

Vaeyens, R., Güllich, Warr, C. R., & Philippaerts, R. (2009). Talent identification and promotion programmes of Olympic athletes. *Journal of Sports Science*, *27*(13), 1367–1380.

Van de Vliet, P., Van Biesen, D., & Vanlandewijck, Y. C. (2008). Athletic identity and self-esteem in Flemish athletes with a disability. *European Journal of Adapted Physical Activity*, *1*(1), 9–21.

10

COACHING, TALENT IDENTIFICATION AND TALENT DEVELOPMENT IN PARA SPORT: DEVELOPING THE FIELD

Robert Townsend and Olivia Clare
Practitioner Commentary: Graeme Maw

Introduction

Interest in Para sport – from both scholars and practitioners – continues to gain considerable momentum. The result of this heightened attention to Para sport is the 'hypervisibility' of disability in elite sport and the increased focus on the athletic potential and performances of Para athletes[1] (Townsend et al., 2018). Against this background, there has been a clear shift towards the development of national sports policies and the distribution of funds, resources and support are targeted at providing accessible and progressive opportunities for disabled people to participate, compete and perform in sport. Naturally accompanying the rise of the profile and popularity of elite disability sport is a critical focus on developing high quality coaches in these contexts (Douglas, 2020).

Coaching was outlined over 30 years ago by DePauw (1986) alongside a number of research priorities for Para sport. However, relative to the literature on coaching in non-disabled contexts, research on coaching in Para sport is underdeveloped (Townsend et al., 2016). This is an important oversight, as coaches are positioned as crucial to athlete development, and evidence suggests that coaching Para athletes places demands on the skills and knowledge of coaches beyond that usually outlined in non-disabled contexts (Burkett, 2013; Douglas, 2020; Townsend et al., 2016). Furthermore, coaches are considered one of the main stakeholders of the Para athletes' pathways, from the beginning to the end of their careers (Patatas et al., 2020). Yet, the types of coach development support for coaches operating in Para sport is highly variable, with disability often absent from national governing body coach development provision, or 'added on' as

DOI: 10.4324/9781003184430-10

short-term, episodic training programmes (Townsend et al., 2021). This lack of coach education is compounded by limited research insight into the landscape of Para sport coaching informing new and innovative methods of supporting coaches. Therefore, considering the growth in Para sport and the corresponding awareness of the need to build performance pathways for Para athletes (Douglas, 2020) it is necessary to carefully examine the role, practice and function of coaches in talent identification and development pathways. This serves a dual purpose. First, exploring coaching in TID pathways can contribute to the expansion and clarification of evidence-based models of Para sport athlete development – something that is desperately needed (Baker et al., 2017; Patatas et al., 2020). Second, these insights are useful for sports organisations wishing to increase the levels of support and training for the Para sport coaching workforce, an issue that researchers continue to highlight (see Townsend & Cushion, 2021).

The purpose of this chapter is to provide some brief insight and stimulate critical discussion of the contribution of coaches and coaching to talent identification and development (henceforth TID) in Para sport. While it is generally agreed that coaches are involved and highly influential in talent identification it is rarely their primary responsibility, with the task of identifying talent devolved to 'talent scouts' or their equivalents within different sports. Particularly within high performance domains, coaches' roles are primarily focused on the development of athletes already identified and selected into performance programmes, what might be termed talent 'confirmation'. With this in mind, there is a paucity of research looking at the role, practice and function of coaches in TID in Para sport, where talent pathways are often less well-established and therefore there may be some 'blurring' of roles across talent identification and talent confirmation. This chapter is a modest attempt to consider 'where we are at'; that is, highlight the key gaps in research with a view to establishing some productive lines of inquiry for coaching researchers interested in talent identification and development. Before we turn our attention to the role and function of coaches, however, it is worth situating coaches within the Para sport TID context.

The Para sport TID landscape

Understanding the developmental pathways of athletes is of paramount importance to ensuring coaches are able to effectively apply their knowledge and practice to bring about positive athlete outcomes. The identifying features of successful TID pathways in non-disabled sport are well established relative to Para sport contexts. Research has highlighted that sustained financial support for athletes, the development of specialist facilities, the provision of sports science and medicine services, a large pool of athletes, well-developed competition structures, and access to high-quality coaching (cf. Green & Houlihan, 2005) are key characteristics of elite sport performance pathways. In Para sport, however, these features tend to be noticeably absent (Taylor et al., 2014). As such, it may be assumed that there is no universal model for para athlete development and it can be best understood as 'non-linear' and 'fluid' (Patatas et al., 2020, 2022). The developmental journey can be thus divided into six intersecting phases: (1) Attraction; (2) Retention; (3) Competition; (4) Talent Identification and Talent Development; (5) Elite; and (6) (voluntary and involuntary) Retirement. A key point of difference between Para sport and non-disabled sport is that the establishment of the Para sport 'pathways' has followed a somewhat unique and fragmented trajectory, with organised disability sports programmes having been historically provided by separate disability sport organisations. Often, these organisations are heavily dependent on government or state funding, and as such are more interested in addressing issues of social inclusion, physical (in)activity and community participation, rather than elite sport development (Houlihan & Chapman, 2017).

However, as the growth in profile and exposure of Para sport increases, a trajectory towards elitism necessitates some organisations adopting elite development strategies and establishing clear performance pathways for Para athletes, either in a decentralised programme under the umbrella of a sports governing body (Wareham et al., 2017) or in a separate disability sport organisation. As such, some sports are heavily reliant on resource sharing as part of a broader mainstreaming or integration agenda with sports governing bodies (Houlihan & Chapman, 2017; Kitchin & Howe, 2014; Thomas & Smith, 2009). As part of this resource sharing, research has identified considerable potential for coaches in non-disabled and Para sport contexts to develop knowledge sharing communities (Duarte et al., 2020). With this in mind, it is worth outlining the unique features of coaches' practices within Para sport in order to better 'bridge the gap' between coaching in non-disabled and Para sport performance pathways. Doing so can go some way to ensuring TID environments better reflect the demands of Para sport while retaining a high-performance or performance development objective.

'The same but different': Coaching in Para sport

Research continues to position coaches and coaching as crucial to the delivery of Para sport performance programmes (Allan et al., 2020; DePauw & Gavron, 1991; Townsend et al., 2016, 2018). Indeed, research interest in Para sport coaching has a long history, but more recently has gained significant momentum. For example, research has explored the role and characteristics of coaches in this context (DePauw & Gavron, 1991), the development of coaches' knowledge (Duarte & Culver, 2014; Taylor et al., 2014), and athletes' perceptions of effective coaching practices (Alexander et al., 2020). These developments have provided much needed insight into the Para sport coaching context, highlighting areas of commonality (Douglas, 2020) with non-disabled contexts, while illustrating the unique features of coaches' practices within Para sport. Research has further highlighted an entrenched 'fear of the unknown' – characterised by a hesitancy or a lack of confidence to work with Para athletes (Townsend et al., 2017; Wareham et al. 2017) a situation that underlines the necessity for coach education to better prepare coaches to work with Para athletes (Townsend et al., 2018). In this context, however, coaching and TID is relatively underdeveloped in existing research, meaning that the evidence base for organisations and practitioners to draw upon to better support athletes in their trajectories through Para sport is limited.

Coaching and talent identification: Through a disability lens

Coaches are generally assumed to have a level of influence and power in TID settings (see Christensen & Henriksen, 2013; Rynne et al., 2017). Existing research has highlighted how in many Para sport pathways coaches exert significant influence on the development of TID initiatives; recruiting athletes into performance programmes through personal networks, outlining performance benchmarks and standards and developing Para-specific resources and guidelines for coaches (Radtke &Doll-Tepper, 2014). Indeed, at all levels of disability sport, coaches are well placed to provide individualised, personal support to enhance athletes' opportunities for, access to, and participation in, sport (Townsend et al., 2018). However, research consistently points to limited investment, training and support for coaches working with Para athletes (Townsend et al., 2018, 2021). This is particularly the case for coaches working at the 'lower' end of the coaching pathway, for example in community sports programmes and clubs.

So, while coaching and talent identification in Para sport is an emerging area of research (Radtke & Doll-Tepper, 2014), in contrast, there is a significant body of literature in talent identification in non-disabled contexts (see, for example, Collins & Bailey, 2013). Given that in Para sport contexts, coaches tend to operate according to principles, theories and concepts developed through experience in non-disabled sport (see Townsend et al., 2018) it is necessary to consider critically the contextual nuances of Para sport that can influence coaches' knowledge-practices in TID settings. Furthermore, this may help to avoid the simplistic transfer of non-disabled TID principles to Para sport contexts (Baker et al., 2017; Dehghansai et al., 2021).

There are two assumptions that underpin the process of talent identification in non-disabled performance pathways. It is worth considering these assumptions and their relevance in Para sport. The first is that coaches need to deliberately reduce the number of athletes they work with and limit it to 'the best' of a particular pool of athletes, typically during developmental or adolescent stages (cf. Rynne et al., 2017). One main factor that influences talent identification is that the 'pipeline' of athletes in disability sport is often much smaller, with athletes with impairments engaging in sport at various developmental stages and for whom access to sport is restricted by complex and multifaceted barriers to participation, which, by default, narrow the talent pool. Furthermore, research continues to highlight the constraints associated with coaching in Para sport contexts, including limited financial support resulting in fewer coaching and support staff, as well as a lack of coaching and training resources and equipment which may further reduce the capacity of a Para sport program (Taylor et al., 2014).

Arguably, existing research has limited itself to the pragmatic features of talent identification in Para sport (Baker et al., 2017), that – while providing valuable insight – neglect the social and cultural factors that influence these processes, and in particular overlooking the issue of power (Christensen & Henriksen, 2013). Coaches exert significant power and influence in Para sport, and talent identification involves a process of inclusion and exclusion (Christensen & Henriksen, 2013) with heavily displaced power relations between coaches and athletes. Importantly this process of TID serves to structure the field of Para sport, providing opportunities for some, but not all. As such, for Para athletes the process of talent identification in Para sport is closely linked to notions of access and equity, where the recognition of talented athletes is constrained by a number of factors, what Thomas (1999) referred to as the *imposed* social restrictions constituting disability. These might include a lack of willing coaches (Wareham et al., 2017) placing active restrictions on the number of athletes that have the opportunity to participate and compete. Another important consideration is how coaches understand disability, and how they are able to reconcile notions of 'talent' with culturally embedded, often negative, ideas about disability. Further, factors related to access heavily influence talent identification, such as the accessibility of facilities, the visibility of programmes and competitive pathways, individuals' ability to sustain participation, and individual impairment effects (e.g., pain, fatigue when competing). Finally, there are factors embedded within the organisational structure of performance sport, including key decision-making considerations such as classification and eligibility, as well as secondary concerns such as how many athletes the organisation can afford to support. Thus, coaches can act as interpersonal mediators, or more simply as 'gatekeepers' to elite sport and by inference TID pathways. How coaches are implicated in 'access work' then, is of prime importance to the study of TID in Para sport.

The second assumption from the broader TID research is that coaches draw on sets of principles, constructs or practice theories that they apply – implicitly and explicitly – to talent identification, and which inform their judgments about 'talented' athletes and their potential (Collins & Bailey, 2013; Roberts et al., 2019). These concepts are often influenced heavily by the disciplines of psychology, physiology and skill acquisition, providing a level of perceived instrumentalism to talent identification (cf. Collins & Bailey, 2013) and foregrounding coaches' expert application of knowledge. When we consider that coaches tend to draw often implicitly on culturally embedded ideas about disability in their practices (Townsend et al., 2018), it is necessary to examine closely the principles of differentiation that coaches use to identify talented athletes. The socialisation of athletes into Para sport begins with the introduction into and acquisition of accepted norms, values and discourses framing performance sport. So too with coaches, where cultural discourses about disability circulate and become embedded within elite sport environments, directing coaches' values and preferences within a particular coaching sub-culture. As such, exploring the principles and discourses used to construct 'talent' in Para sport is an important addition to the Para coaching literature, in particular, how coaches reconcile notions of 'talent' with culturally-embedded notions of disability.

A number of scholars (Christensen, 2009; Christensen & Henriksen, 2013) have raised questions about the social construction of the 'coach's eye', a metaphor designed to challenge the assumption that talent identification is solely 'based on rational or objective processes' (Rynne et al., 2017, p. 288). While the more systematic processes underpinning TID in disability sport are well developed (see, for example Dehghansai et al., 2020 for an excellent overview), the 'experience-based judgements' of coaches which characterise talent identification (Christensen, 2009, p. 367) are less well understood. This is important when we consider that disability itself is constructed through culture, attitudes and relationships and it is worth asking critical questions about the knowledge that coaches draw upon in identifying 'talented' athletes. This is particularly the case when the dominant frame of reference for understanding disability in domains such as medicine, education and indeed sport is the medical model (Townsend et al., 2016).

The implication of the dominance of the medical model in TID is that the recognition of talent is primarily based on the measurement of psychological, physical and physiological attributes (Dehghansai et al., 2021), particularly when those attributes are likely to translate into a favourable classification (Radtke & Doll-Tepper, 2014; Patatas et al., 2020) thus placing the athlete in contention to medal or succeed at elite competition

(Dehghansai et al., 2021). Classification is a complex and problematic practice embedded within Para sport. A key function of the coach in Para sport pathways is to identify athletes that are classifiable, and thus eligible for elite competition (Patatas et al., 2020). While classification is a necessary taxonomy for organisation competition and ensuring – inasmuch as it is possible – fairness (Howe, 2008), *eligibility for* and the *process of* classification itself places limits on who can participate in disability sport, on what basis, and which other athletes can participate (Howe, 2008; Hammond et al., 2019). Thus, classification 'plays an essential role in all phases of Para athletes' pathways' (Patatas et al., 2020, p. 945) and coaches require a working knowledge of classification as poor judgement of classification potential can result in the omission or deselection of athletes into funded programmes (Radtke & Doll-Tepper, 2014).

The extent to which coaches are supported to navigate classification is inconsistent, with Radtke and Doll-Tepper (2014) illustrating how coaches working in 'grassroots' sport often lacked expertise in classifying athletes. More concerningly, recent research has highlighted how an athlete's classification directly influences how prepared coaches are to include athletes in their programmes (see Hammond et al., 2019). Disability (and impairment) therefore are central to conversations related to TID in disability sport (Dehghansai et al., 2021), particularly when coaches' decision-making centres on allocating time and limited resources to athletes whose performance (and medal) potential cannot be assumed (Christensen & Henriksen, 2013). As such, there is a dominant knowledge system in Para sport that ensures coaches identify athletes that are 'hyper-able' where an athlete's impairment is a primary indicator of athletic performance, 'talent' and, thus, their 'medal potential'. Considering the broader IPC rhetoric about driving cultural shifts in how disability is understood in the wider culture, it is worth questioning the extent that coaches' TID practices simply reproduce the 'hyper-able' Para athlete. On the other hand, while it has been argued recently that there are lower levels of representation of athletes from lower classifications or those with higher support needs in performance pathways, if impairment and function is considered a primary determinant of medal potential there is a need to understand instances of coaches deliberately targeting athletes from lower classification. In this case, medal potential may be easier to guarantee where the competition pool is significantly reduced.

A primary driver of medical model practices in TID is the concept of ableism. Ableism contends that there is a tendency for coaches to adopt notions of 'able-bodiedness' as the frame of reference against which to assess ability and – by extension – which athletes are talented. This perspective is accentuated through coaching discourses and practices that are based uncritically on non-disabled elite sport (Townsend et al., 2018) and are designed to render disability 'invisible' (DePauw, 1997) through the proliferation of athlete first discourses (Townsend & Cushion, 2021). While seemingly progressive, ableism provides an ideological framework for coaches in which athletes and their performances are assessed by how closely their performances approximate to non-disabled athletes, and where athletes are judged on how closely they 'fit in' to existing TID structures (Hammond et al., 2019).

In connecting with concepts such as ableism, researchers are better positioned to question the practices and conditions that frame coaching in TID pathways, and in particular to challenge its assumed coherency and rationality. More research therefore is required to shed light on talent identification in Para sport, in particular research that unpacks coaches' beliefs about talent, examining how 'talented athlete' ideals are reconciled with cultural notions of disability that are framed by ableism. As such, this may provide a fruitful line of scholarship while providing some valuable insight for practitioners embedded within Para sport performance pathways (Dehghansai et al., 2021), as well as having clear implications for the education and support of coaches in these domains.

Coach and athlete development: A brief look around

There is an emerging body of research pertaining to the development of Para athletes (Dehghansai et al., 2020, 2021; Patatas et al., 2020, 2022). This research has been extremely valuable in distinguishing Para athletes' developmental trajectories apart from non-disabled models of athlete development, highlighting the uniqueness and complexity of Para sport. As such, it is worth briefly reflecting on the existing research in Para athlete development in order to signal potential ways forward for coaching research.

Without wishing to reiterate the point too much, it is generally assumed that it is essential to match talented athletes with talented coaches to optimise athlete development (Baker et al., 2017). However in Para sport both coaching and athlete development research has, arguably, progressed in relative isolation. In existing athlete development research coaches and their knowledge, practice and function are subsumed within athlete development models – where their efficacy is assumed rather than evidenced. In practice, however, athlete development is interwoven in the daily knowledge-practices of coaches. Coaches' learning in Para sport has been shown to be anchored entirely in their day-to-day experiences – a process of 'trial and error', cherry picking coaching approaches and practice frameworks based on a self-referential process of 'what works' in non-disabled contexts (Townsend et al., 2018). Surprisingly little research has actively sought to understand the formation and application of coaches' knowledge or the impact of coaching practice on athlete development. Perhaps due to the (relative) lack of research on Para athlete development providing direction for coaches, a common situation is that coaches in Para sport tend to adapt existing models and ideas from non-disabled sports contexts and apply them to Para sport contexts (Baker et al., 2017). The application and transfer of athlete development principles by coaches then is a concern, where it may be assumed that the developmental trajectories are the same for both non-disabled and Para athletes. This is problematic, considering the nature and impact of impairment on an athlete's physical maturation, function, movement patterns, body composition, and responsiveness to training (Baker et al., 2017). Furthermore, there are additional considerations when providing 'wrap around' support and care for Para athletes, as Para athletes may experience different social, emotional, and cognitive developmental patterns to non-disabled athletes. More critically, this suggests a degree of ableism underpinning athlete development principles in Para sport which has implications for athlete welfare.

Related to the process of athlete development is the notion of 'talent transfer'. Drawn from research in non-disabled sport (MacNamara & Collins, 2015), talent transfer involves the targeted transfer and 'fast tracking' of an athlete from one sports programme to another to increase the chances of success. In talent transfer initiatives, coaches have been positioned as crucial to their success, in particular developing individualised programmes (MacNamara & Collins, 2015) to enable successful transfer between disciplines. As such, this aspect of talent development in Para sport warrants further attention, particularly due to the lower numbers of participants in talent pathways. For example, talent transfer can either be athlete-initiated whereby athletes may be looking for a new challenge, or coach-led, through the 'shoulder-tapping' of Para athletes from another sports programme. This transfer between sports may increase chances of success by achieving a favourable classification or through maximising the developmental investment made in current athletes. Talent transfer may also be achieved through the ethically dubious targeting of rehabilitation facilities for athletes following traumatic injury or illness (Radtke & Doll-Tepper, 2014) – particularly those with a background in sport – and raising awareness of sports opportunities available (Patatas et al., 2020).

Finally, there is an emerging research area that suggests that some Para athletes experience an accelerated and variable developmental trajectory (Dehghansai et al., 2021) compared to able bodied athletes. This can refer to instances whereby their 'talent transfer' between participation (e.g., clubs, schools) and performance domains is faster than usual. While this is an interesting area for future inquiry it is worth also considering the impact of such trajectories on the learning and development of coaches. With a lack of visible and coherent developmental pathways for coaches in Para sport, it is not uncommon for Para athletes to work with 'personal' coaches that stay with them as they move through the performance pathway (Radtke & Doll-Tepper, 2014). These coaches generally are not employed by the sports governing body or federation, but may receive remuneration as long as the governing body of the sport is satisfied with their performance, or are paid by the athletes who are funded by the governing body. As Townsend et al. (2021) argue, as coaches switch between domains, greater demands are placed on their skills, knowledge and expertise, particularly where coaching domains exacerbate differences in athlete development (e.g., inexperienced coaches working in high-performance domains). Further research is required to understand the longitudinal impact of coaches' accelerated journeys through Para sport.

Coach education is an emerging topic in Para sport. It has been argued elsewhere that coach education requires a major shift to accommodate knowledge about disability (see Townsend et al., 2018), and understandably, for sports governing bodies there is an immediate question of 'what to do' to support the development of Para coaches. Existing coach development models tend to rely heavily on the integration of psychological and bio-scientific discourses as a principle means of informing coaching practice (Townsend et al., 2018). These approaches emphasise a technical language and specialised body of knowledge specific to impairment driving practice. The logic underpinning this approach holds that if coaches can be exposed to the processes and features of impairment, they are better equipped to develop specific interventions (Townsend et al., 2017). While we know that impairment presents a direct consideration for coaches in practice, there is a danger in coach education to prescribe coaching approaches based solely on impairment-specific information.

At this stage there are no 'clear cut' answers for improving the level of support for coaches' learning in Para sport, particularly because delivering optimal coach education programmes incorporates a level of complexity not currently observed in Para coaching. For example, there is a need to base coach education on evidence-based approaches to professional learning combined with a framework for understanding disability that centralises the reflective focus on the knowledge, practice and skills of coaches, as well as an understanding of impairment that recognises its impact on athletes' developmental trajectories, while not being the dominating feature. While a social relational model has been proposed elsewhere (see Townsend et al., 2018), one productive line of inquiry established due to the lack of consensus on optimal frameworks for athlete and coach development in Para sport is the utilisation of Newell's (1986) constraints-based framework as both a *model of* athlete development and *model for* coaches to consider (see Baker et al., 2017; Dehghansai et al., 2021). This model emphasises the need for coaches to optimise athletes' functional ability rather than manage their lack of function and is considered a useful tool in informing coaches' decision-making. The evidence base is emerging, and so there remain questions about the translation of this model into existing coach education structures as well as its reception and application by coaches in talent development contexts. Indeed, researchers may wish to explore, combine and extend both the social relational model and a constraints-based framework in a grounded exploration of coaching in TID pathways, as a means of extending scholarship in Para sport and informing coach development.

Key questions and considerations

A cursory assessment of the emerging body of research in Para sport reveals a range of theoretical perspectives and insights into talent identification and athlete development, as well as a number of opportunities for research. Within Para sport performance pathways coaches are positioned as a major stakeholder, applying considerable influence over talent identification and athlete development. Despite this, an in-depth understanding of the coaching process – inclusive of talent identification and development – in Para sport is lacking. As such, it is difficult to build shared consensus or provide direction for coaches and practitioners in these contexts. Consequently, TID practices are often based on the application and translation of non-disabled principles or coaches are left to operate without reference to a framework or model for best practice. Understandably, this has led researchers – predominantly housed in the discipline of skill acquisition – to promote a framework based on ecological dynamics to enhance coaching practice in TID. While a useful conceptual development in Para sport, arguably we do not know enough about coaching generally, nor in Para sport environments, to prescribe coaching approaches. This can risk oversimplifying a phenomenon, which can limit the conceptual development of coaching and reproduce certain understandings of coaching in Para sport that align with a dominant psychological paradigm.

A targeted research agenda, developed in partnership with organisations responsible for TID in Para sport then seems a reasonable area for future development. In particular, we encourage understandings of coaching to be grounded *in context*, and as such require connections to broader ideas in the study of disability. For example, in this chapter we have highlighted potential connections between talent identification practices and notions of access and equity. This is a significant conceptual development, because *recognition of* talent is predicated on the assumption that talented athletes have navigated a series of exclusionary barriers to participate in sport. The role of the coach in facilitating access and opportunity requires further research. Furthermore, we have highlighted the need to understand the constructed nature of the principles that coaches draw upon to recognise 'talent' as it intersects with disability.

Finally, the training of coaches is considered one of the most pressing matters in sustaining and improving the quality of sports provision for Para athletes (Townsend et al., 2017; Townsend et al., 2018). The extent to which coaches are supported within TID environments is not clear, but a broader assessment of the coach development literature suggests an absence of disability-specific content in formalised coach education programmes and inconsistency in the availability and impact of disability-specific coach education provision. As such, with recent moves toward integration in Para sport there is an opportunity to seek alternatives to 'standard', formalised coach education programmes as sources of professional development (Duarte et al., 2020) for coaches. In particular, approaches in which disability is infused throughout the routines and curricula may be of particular benefit for coaches in Para sport performance pathways (Townsend et al., 2018). Researchers also have a crucial role to play in reforming coach education, where disabled people must be included in a partnership model that centralises and values disability-specific knowledge to inform the development of educational programmes, resources and content for coaches. Currently, it is possible that practice is moving faster in Para sport than research, and so partnership models between practitioners and researchers is required to ensure innovation is empirically-grounded and evidence-led.

Concluding thoughts

This chapter has given insight into the current 'lay of the land' in Para sport TID focusing in particular on the role of coaches. It has highlighted the lack of research situated in Para sport contexts and, therefore, the over-reliance on research in non-disabled sport to bridge the gap. Translation from non-disabled sport practices results in practices influenced by ableism that do not acknowledge the unique context in which Para sport unfolds. Para athletes face an array of barriers that differ considerably from those faced by non-disabled athletes as well as differing needs, and TID practices must reflect this. Furthermore, it is not uncommon for community-based coaches to find themselves suddenly (and sometimes unexpectedly) coaching a Paralympic athlete and the lack of clear, coherent development pathways for coaches alongside a scarcity of best practice frameworks to draw on may limit athlete development. The conceptual development of Para sport scholarship is crucial to inform practice, where targeted research agendas across coach and athlete development is needed to inform organisations responsible for Para sport performance pathways. Developing guiding principles for coaches and effective coach development pathways from these insights is necessary to ensure Para athletes have the best chance of progressing successfully along performance pathways.

Acknowledgements

Thanks must go to Dr Graeme Maw for providing valuable feedback on a draft of this chapter and the encouragement of the ideas herein.

Practitioner commentary

Coaching, talent identification and talent development form a fascinating landscape in Paralympic sport, as they do in Olympic sport, and as suggested in the chapter, there is indeed a paucity of published information in the former compared to the latter. At the same time, however, there is growing practical involvement and knowledge in Para sport, with this evolution potentially progressing well ahead of publication; our practice-based evidence is ploughing a path for research to follow.

The Tokyo 2020 Paralympic Games saw 162 nations compete in 22 sports, with a record 86 nations winning medals. For each of these nations' sportsmen and women, coaching was naturally a key component to their development and success.

While coaching in Para sport contexts may not have the body of literature that coaching in Olympic sports has, the fundamental purpose and principles of coaching remain the same – to help an individual to develop to the best of their ability. This is true in sport, business and education. The focus is therefore on individualisation, working with an athlete's abilities and limitations, the same way any expert coach views their charge.

In my experience, this individualisation offers the best examples of coaching, with the coach's problem-solving skills to the fore. Increasingly, and encouraged by the trend towards integrated sports bodies – coaches work simultaneously and exchangeably across Para and Olympic pathways. Coaching practice therefore remains the same, and it is arguably the technical knowledge to be added (e.g., how do limb deficiencies impact training tolerance or how do intellectual impairments impact communication?). The scientific, rather than coaching community, perhaps needs to catch up.

With this increasing cross-over, associated funding and growth in the Para sport movement, it is also important to consider our language. Para sport is no longer fringe! Indeed, in New Zealand 24% of the population identify as having some form of disability. Of course not everyone will be eligible for Paralympic sport, but shows the likelihood of inclusive sports coaches working with athletes with impairments. For reference (and aligned with this text), Sport New Zealand's position is that 'disabled' refers to a person's environmental barriers rather than their impairment, and with close to NZ\$12 m being invested by the government in the next three years, Para and disability sport is certainly more mainstream than many niche sports.

Unfortunately, one of the barriers encountered by coaches in furthering Para sport growth remains uncertainty – even fear – and a lack of confidence in providing initial support. Townsend and Clare rightly point out the role of ableist language in perpetuating this fear. However, emphasising the coaches' role in talent identification may also limit access: If the talent pathway is the primary purpose for Para sport, then the gateway will be narrow. This is a truism in all sport, and positioning the coach as central to talent identification (aka 'selection') belies those fundamental principles of true coaching.

Long live coaches who aim to develop all individuals, and the growing knowledge, such as this chapter, to increase inclusion.

Note

1 Given our focus on disability sport with a high-performance or performance development objective, for clarity, we will use Para sport and para athletes throughout. However, we align fundamentally with the social model of disability, where we acknowledge that disability is an accumulation of oppressive practices and discourses that marginalise and exclude people with impairments. At the same time, we acknowledge and support the preference by some for person-first terms.

References

Alexander, D., Bloom, G. A., & Taylor, S. (2020). Female Paralympic athlete views of effective and ineffective coaching practices. *Journal of Applied Sport Psychology*, *32*(1), 48–63.

Allan, V., Blair Evans, M., Latimer-Cheung, A. E., & J. Côté, J. (2020). From the athletes' perspective: A social-relational understanding of how coaches shape the disability sport experience. *Journal of Applied Sport Psychology*, *32*(6), 546–564.

Baker, J., Lemez, S., Van Neutegem, A. & Wattie, N. (2017). Talent development in Parasport. In J. Baker, S. Cobley, J. Schorer and N. Wattie (Eds.) *Routledge handbook of talent identification and development in Sport* (pp. 432–442). New York: Rouledge.

Burkett, B. (2013). Coaching athletes with a disability. In P. Potrac, W. Gilbert and J. Denison (Eds.) *Routledge handbook of sports coaching* (pp. 196–209). New York: Routledge.

Christensen, M. K. (2009). "An eye for talent": Talent identification and the "practical sense" of top-level soccer coaches. *Sociology of Sport Journal*, *26*, 365–382.

Christensen, M. K. & Henriksen, K. (2013). Coaches and talent identification. In P. Potrac, W. Gilbert, & J. Denison (Eds.) *Routledge handbook of sports coaching* (pp. 160–171). New York: Routledge.

Collins, D. & Bailey, R. (2013). Scienciness and the allure of secondhand strategy in talent identification and development. *International Journal of Sport Policy and Politics*, 5(2), 183–191.

Dehghansai, N., Lemez, S., Wattie, N., Pinder, R. A., & Baker, J. (2020). Understanding the development of elite Parasport athletes using a constraint-led approach: Considerations for coaches and practitioners. *Frontiers in Psychology*, 11, 502981.

Dehghansai, N., Pinder, R. A. & Baker, J. (2021). Looking for a golden needle in the haystack: Perspectives on talent identification and development in Paralympic sport. *Frontiers in Sports and Active Living*, 3, 635977.

DePauw, K. P. (1986). Toward progressive inclusion and acceptance: Implications for physical education. *Adapted Physical Activity Quarterly*, 3, 1–6.

DePauw, K. P. (1997). The (in)visibility of disAbility: Cultural contexts and sporting bodies. *Quest*, 49(4), 416–430.

DePauw, K. P., & Gavron, S. J. (1991). Coaches of athletes with disabilities. *The Physical Educator*, 48, 33–40.

Douglas, S. (2020). Better coaching, better athletes: Developing quality coaches of athletes with impairments. In. B. Callary & B. Gearity (Eds.) *Coach education and development in sport: Instructional strategies* (pp. 226–236). New York: Routledge.

Duarte, T. & Culver, D. M. (2014). Becoming a coach in developmental adaptive sailing: A lifelong learning approach. *Journal of Applied Sport Psychology*, 26(4), 441–456.

Duarte, T., Culver, D. M., & Paquette, K. (2020). Mapping Canadian wheelchair curling coaches' development: A landscape metaphor for a systems approach. *International Sport Coaching Journal*, 7(2), 117–126.

Green, M., & Houlihan, B. (2005). *Elite sport development: Policy learning and political priorities*. London: Routledge

Hammond, A., Jeanes, R., Penney, D., & Leahy, D. (2019). 'I feel we are inclusive enough': Examining swimming coaches' understandings of inclusion and disability. *Sociology of Sport Journal*, 36(4), 311–321.

Houlihan, B. & Chapman, P. (2017) Talent identification and development in elite youth disability sport. *Sport in Society*, 20(1), 107–125.

Howe, P. D. (2008). The tail is wagging the dog: Body culture, classification and the paralympic movement. *Ethnography*, 9(4), 499–517.

Kitchin, P. J., & Howe, P. D. (2014). The mainstreaming of disability cricket in England and Wales: Integration 'one game' at a time. *Sport Management Review*, 17, 65–77.

MacNamara, A. & Collins, D. (2015). Second chances: Investigating athletes' experiences of talent transfer. *Plos One*, 10(11), 1–13.

Patatas, J. M., De Bosscher, V., Derom, I. & De Rycke, J. (2020) Managing parasport: An investigation of sport policy factors and stakeholders influencing para-athletes' career pathways. *Sport Management Review*, 23(5), 937–951.

Patatas, J. M., De Bosscher, V., Derom, I., & Winckler, C. (2022). Stakeholders' perceptions of athletic career pathways in Paralympic sport: From participant to excellence. *Sport in Society*, 25(2), 299–320.

Radtke, S., & Doll-Tepper, G. (2014). *A cross-cultural comparison of talent identification and development in Paralympic Sports*. Cologne: Sportverlag.

Roberts, A. H., Greenwood, D. A., Stanley, M., Humberstone, C., Iredale, F. & Raynor, A. (2019). Coach knowledge in talent identification: A systematic review and meta-synthesis. *Journal of Science and Medicine in Sport*, *22*(10), 1163–1172.

Rynne, S. B., Crudgington, B., Dickinson, R. K. & Mallett, C. J. (2017). On the (potential) value of coaches. In J. Baker, S. Cobley, J. Schorer & N. Wattie (Eds.) *Routledge handbook of talent identification and development in sport* (pp. 285–300), Routledge.

Taylor, S. L., Werthner, P., & Culver, D. M. (2014). A case study of a parasport coach and a life of learning. *International Journal of Sport Coaching*, *1*(3), 127–138.

Thomas, C. (1999). *Female forms: Experiencing and understanding disability*. Oxfordshire: Open University Press.

Thomas, N. & Smith, A. (2009). *Disability, sport and society: An introduction*. London: Routledge.

Townsend, R. C., & Cushion, C. J. (2021). Put that in your fucking research: Reflexivity, ethnography and disability sport coaching. *Qualitative Research*, *21*(2), 251–267.

Townsend, R. C., Cushion, C. J., & Smith. B. (2017). A social-relational analysis of an impairment-specific mode of coach education. *Qualitative Research in Sport, Exercise and Health*, *10*(3), 346–361.

Townsend, R. C., Huntley, T. D., Cushion, C. J., & Fitzgerald. H. (2018). It's not about disability, I want to win as many medals as possible: The social construction of disability in high-performance coaching. *International Review for the Sociology of Sport*, *55*(3), 344–360.

Townsend, R. C., Smith, B., & Cushion, C. J. (2016). Disability sports coaching: Towards a critical understanding. *Sports Coaching Review*, *4*(2), 80–98.

Wareham, Y., Burkett, B., Innes, P., & Lovell, G. (2017). Coaching athletes with disability: Preconceptions and reality. *Sport in Society*, *20*(9), 1185–1202.

11

ROLE OF TECHNOLOGY IN ATHLETE ASSESSMENT

Sonja de Groot, Barry Mason, and Riemer Vegter
Practitioner Commentary: David Haydon

Introduction

Many factors play a role in talent development. Factors related to both the athlete (i.e., rate of learning, training and maturation of anthropometric, physiological, technical, tactical and psychological skills), the environment (i.e., opportunities created by parents, trainers, coaches, and the competition structure), along with a component of chance (Elferink-Gemser & Visscher, 2012) – see Figure 11.1.

Progression in Para sport will also be dependent on the task characteristics associated with each sport. In Para Athletics, success in the sprint and field events will largely be determined by physical and technical progress. Other sports, like Wheelchair Fencing, will be strongly underpinned by technical skills. However, in sports such as the wheelchair court sports a large emphasis is placed on tactical awareness which is likely to be the biggest barrier to fast-tracking talented individuals into high-performing athletes. So, talent development is an interplay between the task characteristics, environment and performance characteristics (Figure 11.1).

In this chapter, the focus will be on the role of technology in athlete assessment to support talent development. Therefore, examples of technology for testing and monitoring performance characteristics such as anthropometric, physiological, technical, and tactical skills applicable to adapted sports will be described.

DOI: 10.4324/9781003184430-11

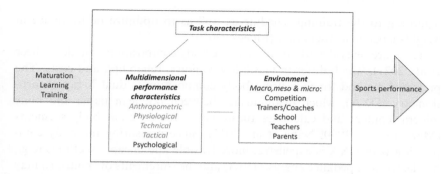

FIGURE 11.1 Adapted version of the (Elferink-Gemser & Visscher, 2012) model showing the development of a talented athlete's sport performance over time with the hypothetical contribution of person-related, task-related, and environmental characteristics to sport performance in talented athletes. The characteristics highlighted in red will be described in this chapter

Technology for testing and monitoring of *anthropometric* characteristics

Anthropometric data are often used for talent identification. Factors such as body mass, height, reaching height, and sitting height are all often thought to be related to performance outcomes in specific contexts. The ability to reach can be dependent upon arm length but also on trunk stability, which is related to the disability of the athlete. Reaching can be measured by, for example, pushing away a tube as far as possible (Kouwijzer et al., 2020) which can be combined with inertial measurement units (IMUs) to measure trunk stability. Sitting height can also be a performance characteristic in some sports; for example, taller players are often thought to have an advantage in Wheelchairheelchair Basketball because their ability to reach higher into the air yields a better chance of shooting over an opponent, rebounding and blocking shorter players' shots.

Body composition can also be more or less important in certain sports and is related to health. For example, in most rolling sports it is favourable to have a low fat mass since it leads to a lower rolling resistance and, therefore, better performance (van der Woude et al., 2001). However, a fat mass that is too low can have a negative effect on health so the body composition should be monitored carefully.

Endurance sport athletes show the lowest body mass from all sports; when comparing different wheelchair sports, the lowest fat mass was found in Para Cycling athletes (12.5 ± 6.5 kg) whereas curling game players showed the highest total fat mass (25.3 ± 4.9 kg) and basketball players showed the highest fat-free mass (Flueck, 2020). It seems worthwhile to track body composition in Para sport athletes to optimize the energy needs regarding to the training schedule as well as to optimize performance in weight-dependent disciplines (Flueck, 2020).

There are several methods to measure body composition (van der Scheer et al., 2021), which differ in feasibility, validity, reliability, and costs. The preferred method for measuring body composition is dual X-ray absorptiometry (DXA), which distinguishes between fat, lean tissue and bone mineral content and calculates those values for different body segments (Mazess et al., 1990; Nana et al., 2015). Since measuring the body composition with DXA is expensive, more feasible and cheaper methods (e.g., bioelectrical impedance analysis (BIA) and measurements of skinfolds) may be preferable. BIA is a non-invasive test in which two electrodes are placed on the athlete's right hand and foot, if applicable, and a weak electric current is sent through the body. However, existing BIA as well as skinfold equations should always be used with caution in Para sport athletes, especially in athletes with substantial body asymmetry (Goosey-Tolfrey et al., 2016), such as those with limb loss, or for athletes with substantial muscle atrophy (Moore et al., 2015).

Another important aspect is monitoring the dietary intake to see whether the athletes' intake balances their needs regarding calories and nutrients. Although various methods are available for gathering dietary data, those based on innovative technologies are particularly promising. With combined cost-effectiveness and ease of use, technologies like mobile phone applications can now optimize tracking of eating occasions and dietary behaviours (Simpson et al., 2017). However, it should be kept in mind that the estimation of energy needs is often based on the general population and is not always applicable to athletes with a disability. People with a spinal cord injury, for example, can have a 25% lower resting energy expenditure than the general population (Buchholz & Pencharz, 2004). Energy expenditure during exercise is also typically reduced in athletes with spinal cord injury between 25–75%, with the greatest energy expenditure reduction in athletes with tetraplegia or those participating in static wheelchair sports (Goosey-Tolfrey et al., 2014). Furthermore, the energy needs and expenditures of individuals with a central neurologic injury, such as cerebral palsy, vary greatly because of the wide range of associated functional impairment related to activities. Inefficiencies in ambulation and the presence of athetosis, spasticity, or ataxia, may all increase energy requirements, while decreased oral motor function may reduce oral intake (Crosland & Boyd, 2014). Consequently, body composition and energy balance (i.e., energy expenditure and intake) should be carefully monitored and individualised for all Para sport athletes during talent development.

Technology for testing and monitoring of *physiological* characteristics

When training for matches and races, normally the first goal is to become as fit as possible. This fitness is often expressed as the anaerobic and aerobic capacity. The anaerobic energy system is important for short-term performance, up to 1–2 minutes, and is most often estimated by the power output generated during a sprint or Wingate test (De Groot et al., 2012). The aerobic energy system reflects the ability to perform dynamic, moderate-to-vigorous intensity exercise with the largest possible muscle mass for prolonged periods of time. Peak oxygen uptake (VO_2peak) and peak aerobic power output have been identified as important descriptors of the aerobic energy system and can be assessed with a graded exercise test until exhaustion (Baumgart et al., 2020; De Groot et al., 2012).

Both anaerobic and aerobic capacity relate to the match and race performance. For example, in an endurance sport like Handcycling (Nevin & Smith, 2020) and Para Triathlon (Stephenson et al., 2020), it was found that anaerobic and aerobic power are highly correlated with race time. Therefore, it is important to measure and monitor the anaerobic and aerobic capacity for designing and evaluating athletes' strength and conditioning programs.

Research under laboratory and field conditions is complementary; the strength of one approach is the weakness of the other (Thompson & Vanlandewijck, 2020). For example, during field-based testing, the athlete can be tested in conditions closer to their performance environment, which results in a higher external validity, yet the changing environmental conditions make standardisation difficult. Control and reliability are both key advantages of laboratory-based testing. With new technologies, Para sport athletes can be tested in a standardized and sport-specific way in this environment. Graded exercise testing on a treadmill (running, wheelchair propulsion), bike ergometer (cycling) or armcrank ergometer (Handcycling) (Figure 11.2, left picture) are now more common ways of testing in Para sport populations. However, Paralympic athletes in sports where propulsion is achieved by using their arms were quite often tested on an armcrank ergometer while a more sport-specific way of testing would be more favorable. For example, Para Ice Hockey players can be tested while sitting in an ice sledge hockey seat during upper-body poling on a Concept2 ski ergometer (Baumgart et al., 2018).

Wheelchair athletes have been tested on treadmills as well as on wheelchair ergometers. The disadvantages of wheelchair ergometers were that they were not always commercially available and often had a fixed, but adjustable, chair (de Klerk et al., 2020). As a result, it is preferred to test athletes using their own equipment to see their real potential within the limits of their disability. With the commercially available Lode Esseda wheelchair

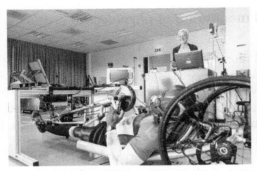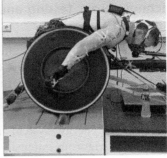

FIGURE 11.2 Specific exercise testing. Left: Exercise test with a handcyclist (photo credit: Marieke van der Heijden); Right: Testing a wheelchair athlete (photo credit: Riemer Vegter)

ergometer (Figure 11.2, right picture), it is possible to test wheelchair athletes in their own chair with a variety of test options such as isometric strength, isokinetic strength and (an)aerobic capacity (de Klerk et al., 2020). Sport-specific testing is important to assess the actual physical fitness and/or physiological attributes to design specifically tailored training protocols and periodization models and to increase the likelihood of success in competition. With sport-specific testing, strengths and weaknesses can be identified and this information can help athletes and coaches to adjust their training programmes.

Technology for testing and monitoring of *technical* characteristics

The technical skills needed for the different Paralympic sports are clearly important. The eventual performance depends on all components of the athlete-assistive device combination, like the use of a lower-limb prosthesis or a wheelchair. This can be subdivided in three major parts (Figure 11.3).

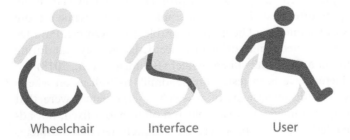

Wheelchair   Interface   User

FIGURE 11.3 Symbolic representation of the components that are important to consider when evaluating the athlete-assistive device combination

First, the athlete will determine the effectiveness of any assistive device, where the appropriate motor skills and physical capacity will determine whether the potential of the device can be used. Second, the assistive device also has its own characteristics like size, mass, stiffness and rolling friction, which need to change in line with the athlete's development. Finally, the connection between the two (i.e., the interface) is defined as how athlete and device are connected and work together. This not only means the literal connection, like a prosthesis socket or wheelchair seat, but also the way they interact in the sense of translating energy from the athlete, via the device, onto the environment, such as the type of knee joint used, or the connection of the hand to the handrim.

Since performance depends on this athlete-assistive device combination, understanding the biomechanics of this combination is key to optimize performance. Therefore, it is not only important to train the physiological capacity of the athlete but also the skill to transfer the power from the hand to the wheelchair rim. Furthermore, an individually optimally tuned interface between the athlete and wheelchair is essential for a good performance. Take, for instance, the skill and interface necessary for coupling the hand with racket to the handrim during Wheelchair Tennis (de Groot et al., 2017). Understanding the interplay between the athlete, interface and wheelchair is very hard and it is not always easy to predict the eventual performance, especially given the variability of human motor control and individual differences in motor skill acquisition. Fortunately, the performance outcomes can be measured and evaluated to optimize an athlete's performance. Below some of the laboratory tools for such measurements are discussed.

Next to overground testing, a treadmill can provide an effective testing environment, where speed and power output can be standardized and controlled. A single axis force transducer can be used to measure the power output through a drag test (Figure 11.4, right). Treadmill inclination or a pulley system can consequently be used to impose the desired power output (Figure 11.4, left). Although treadmills have some advantages, like the need to control left-right power output to go in a straight line, they are more suited for steady-state velocities, rather than acceleration or measurements at very high speeds.

An instrumented roller ergometer (Figure 11.2, right) can be an excellent alternative for sprint testing. Moreover, since the rollers are instrumented, high-frequency continuous measurements of power output can be available in contrast to measurements on a treadmill. These measures can be used to understand wheelchair propulsion biomechanics (Figure 11.5), for example, to evaluate upper-limb asymmetries in wheelchair athletes (Goosey-Tolfrey et al., 2018).

The development of wheelchair ergometers have a long history (de Klerk et al., 2020). Such devices have integrated test protocols to measure isometric

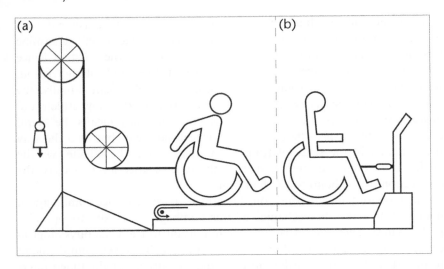

FIGURE 11.4   Experimental setup. Left: To impose the desired power output a pulley-system is attached to the wheelchair on the treadmill. Right: A drag test is performed to determine power output of the user-wheelchair combination

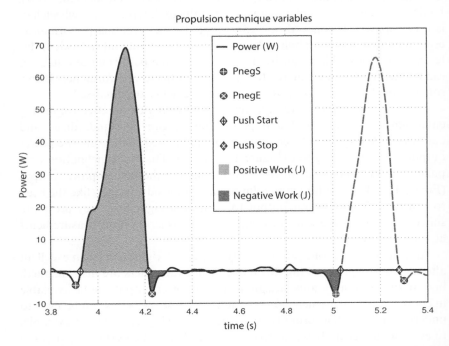

FIGURE 11.5   Illustration of the power output signal from the wheelchair erg-ometer and definition of some wheelchair propulsion outcomes: push time (from push start to push end), cycle time (from push start to push start), and power loss before (PnegS) and after (PnegE) the push time

force and (an)aerobic exercise capacity and thus can be applied for profiling and systematically monitoring the effect of training or changes to the assistive device (Janssen et al., 2021). Furthermore, the wheelchair ergometer can be used during training and direct visual feedback of propulsion technique variables, such as peak force and push time, can be provided to the athlete and coach on a monitor during propulsion to improve specific aspects of wheelchair propulsion (Richter et al., 2011).

In addition to the wheelchair ergometer a number of common measurement tools can be added, such as three-dimensional position registration and electromyography (EMG) to measure muscle activity (Figure 11.6). These more advanced testing setups can be used to answer biomechanical questions about the performance of an athlete (Figure 11.7). Since the upper-limb is a very mobile joint, actually understanding the complex dynamics and kinematics is difficult. The rotator-cuff is actively needed to stabilize the shoulder joint, but also contributes to the force application onto the handrim (Vegter et al., 2015). Moreover, although the task seems fairly constrained, there are still a lot of different degrees of freedom (Mason et al., 2018). The study of Mason et al. (Mason et al., 2018) nicely illustrates the use of these techniques by applying them to understand the role of the scapula and asymmetries in posture and chair positioning in relation to pain and performance in wheelchair athletes.

Developments in technology over recent years have made field-based performance monitoring increasingly accessible to Para sport athletes. IMUs, which typically include accelerometers, gyroscopes and magnetometers, can be

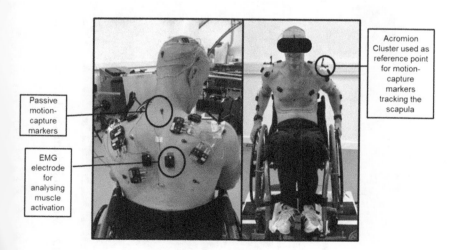

FIGURE 11.6 Wheelchair user showing placement of electromyography (EMG) and passive motion-capture markers to measure muscle activity and movements, respectively (photo credit: Riemer Vegter)

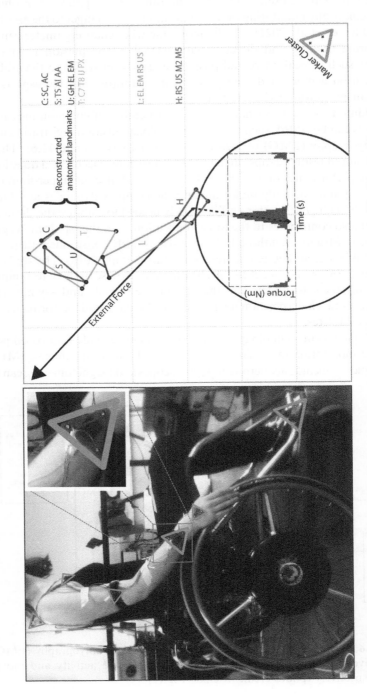

FIGURE 11.7 Measuring kinetics and kinematics and visualizing the outcomes (photo credit: Riemer Vegter)

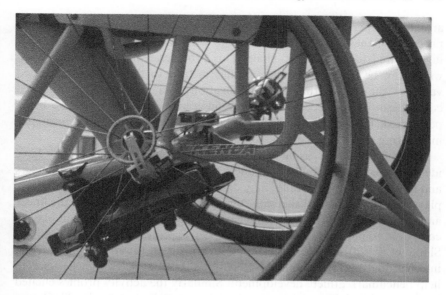

FIGURE 11.8 Inertial Measurement Units (IMUs) attached around the wheel axles and frame (photo credit: Sonja de Groot)

attached around the wheel axis and frame of sports wheelchairs (Figure 11.8). IMUs can provide real-time feedback about linear and rotational acceleration and velocity metrics (van der Slikke et al., 2020). If used longitudinally during standardised field tests, these devices can serve to map out an individuals' progress over time and can help identify the strengths and weaknesses for specific athletes such as left-right symmetry or acceleration from standstill. It provides coaches and practitioners with evidence-based information about the areas that need improving and they can adjust their programmes and practice accordingly to improve these areas. This individualised approach is an important and necessary step when developing talented athletes into high-performance athletes and can serve to expedite this process.

A benefit of IMUs is that they can also be used in non-standardised conditions (i.e., during match-play scenarios) to monitor the performance and progression of athletes during competitive situations. In this type of environment, miniaturised data loggers (MDL) and radio-frequency based indoor tracking systems (ITS) are also viable options for performance monitoring. MDL are wheel-mounted devices that work via reed switch technology and every time a wheel rotates, a magnetic pendulum activates a reed switch to produce a time stamp (Tolerico et al., 2007). With known wheel dimensions, speed and distance metrics can be calculated alongside the number of starts and stops performed. An ITS operates in a very similar way to Global Positioning Systems (GPS), whereby sensors are positioned around the perimeter of an indoor court. After a series of calibration procedures, these sensors communicate wirelessly with small, lightweight tags secured to an athletes' chair. This provides real-time location data, which can be used to calculate similar metrics to the MDL. The added value of the ITS is that because location data is provided, additional context can be acquired about where on court certain activities are being performed (Figure 11.9). This adds a layer of tactical detail to performance monitoring that will be discussed in the next section.

Scientific research using these technologies during match-play have identified the key mobility characteristics of higher ranked teams/players and how their activity profiles may differ compared to lower ranked teams/ players in Wheelchair Basketball, rugby and tennis. For example, the linear and rotational performance of international Wheelchair Basketball players compared to national level players has been captured using IMUs (van der Slikke et al., 2016). These metrics, which were all found to be greater in international players compared to national level athletes, can be used to help benchmark athlete development. Similarly the activity profiles elicited by international Wheelchair Rugby players (Rhodes et al., 2015) and Wheelchair Tennis players (Mason et al., 2020; Sindall et al., 2013) have also been documented using MDL and ITS. This information is incredibly valuable for the development of athletes since it paints a clearer picture of what is required to be a high-performance athlete and if the technology can be used longitudinally, progression can be monitored along the performance pathway. However, accuracy and reliability (MDL) and cost/expertise (ITS) required must always be considered when determining the appropriate technology for the job. IMUs are a cost effective, easy to use, accurate and reliable (van der Slikke et al., 2015) alternative to measure wheelchair performance. Recently, the first attempts have been made to also estimate the power output from IMUs attached to the axle and the wheels (Rietveld et al., 2021). Power output is an objective measure of training load. Nowadays, every elite (hand)cyclist uses a commercially available power meter (Abel et al., 2010; de Groot et al., 2018). In contrast, unfortunately there is not yet a (commercially available) power meter for wheelchair athletes to monitor the external training load next to internal training load measures such as heart rate and rating of perceived exertion.

Tactical

Activity profiles of wheelchair court sport athletes, discussed in the previous section, have also been explored in relation to the outcome of the performance (i.e., winners versus losers) or the ranking/status (high ranked versus low ranked) (Mason et al., 2020; Rhodes et al., 2015; Sindall et al., 2013). These studies have demonstrated that very few differences in activity

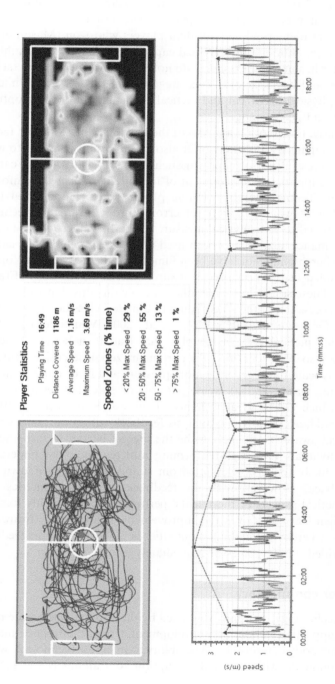

Player Statistics

Playing Time   **16:49**
Distance Covered   **1186 m**
Average Speed   **1.16 m/s**
Maximum Speed   **3.69 m/s**

Speed Zones (% time)

<20% Max Speed   **29 %**
20 - 50% Max Speed   **55 %**
50 - 75% Max Speed   **13 %**
> 75% Max Speed   **1 %**

FIGURE 11.9 Examples of how location data can be used to calculate metrics and to give additional context on where on court certain activities are being performed

profiles existed between high and low-ranked teams in Wheelchair Rugby (Rhodes et al., 2015). Similarly, observations were made in Wheelchair Tennis, where it was revealed that players who lost the match actually performed more high-speed activity than players who won (Mason et al., 2020). Therefore, although the physical capacity of higher ranked athletes may be greater in some contexts, they do not appear reliant on these factors to win games and be successful. This suggests that there is a dynamic interaction of physical, technical and tactical elements that support optimal development and performance.

Subsequently, time motion analysis of the ball handling skills and tactics employed during match-play may offer also an important insight into what determines successful performance in such sports and how these can be monitored to support the development of individuals. This was reinforced in Wheelchair Tennis whereby winning players were characterised by a higher number of winners and fewer errors during a range of technical strokes, compared to any physical measures of performance (Mason et al., 2020). Performance analysis has been used more extensively in Wheelchair Basketball whereby matches have been filmed and the activities performed have been coded using specialised software, such as SportsCode (Francis et al., 2019). These studies have identified specific line-ups that yield higher chances of success than others according to athletes' classification (Francis et al., 2019; Gómez et al., 2015; Molik et al., 2009; Vanlandewijck et al., 2004). Specific tactical patterns of play that lead to a better chance of success have also been identified. In particular, zonal defensive strategies have been advocated to i) generate more pressure and force more turnovers from opposing teams, and ii) create patterns of play that result in more open shots which yield a greater chance of success (Francis et al., 2019).

Subsequently, access to video analysis feedback within the court sports, where tactical awareness is likely to be the biggest barrier to fast-tracking talented individuals into high-performing athletes could be imperative. Learning is likely to be accelerated from simply viewing their own performances back. However, with the feedback of detailed metrics documenting tactical aspects of the talents' performance, it is highly likely to accelerate their learning. Given the improvements in analysis software over recent years, whereby the coding of activities is far easier and the feedback can be provided during games or immediately after.

Practitioner commentary

The use of technology, as rightly discussed by the authors, has a wide range of roles in supporting Para athlete development, from performance analysis to monitoring body composition. The ability to integrate technology within sport environments with minimal disruption to training is the greatest challenge. As researchers and practitioners, we are improving, and this is resulting in greater adoption of technology to support athlete development across the whole pathway.

In practise, one of the more difficult aspects is providing effective feedback. Whether this is technical or tactical, simple improvements in technology (or access to technology and personnel) can change how (e.g., visual in addition to verbal) and when athletes receive feedback. The ability to capture video and replay during training (often in slow motion) allows detailed discussion between the athlete and their coach/support on both technical (e.g., propulsion technique in swimming) and tactical components (e.g., review of planned/structured plays in Wheelchair Rugby). This can be a relatively simple solution in cases where filming and replay is straightforward. However, many training environments, particularly in Para sport contexts, come with their own challenges: minimal support for technology set-up and operation, working with a group of athletes and providing group and individual feedback, or athletes training in remote locations. From my experiences, the more effort associated with using technology, the less likely it is to be implemented and used regularly. The next step for wider adoption of technology discussed by the authors (such as IMUs, MDLs, etc.) requires work to reduce the set-up, operation, and analysis requirements – which is already happening through continued development and research. Semi-permanent installations can help with this where possible, reducing the need for additional support in training sessions. In most cases, the feedback required is not complex – it is the ability to provide clear, key points efficiently and immediately (through available software or expertise if available) that can aid athlete development and support future planning.

Another area in Para sport contexts that has shown considerable progression in recent years is the individual customisation of equipment interfaces. As the authors discuss, interaction between the hand and push rim is critical in ensuring power is transferred to the wheels optimally in wheelchair sports. In Wheelchair Racing, gloves are now being developed from scans of athlete hands and preferred grip positions, with designs then 3D printed specifically for that individual. A similar process can be followed for individualised carbon moulded seats to improve performance, which are lighter, stronger, and more suited to the individual. As technology becomes more widely available, more equipment will continue to be customised for the individual, and for newer athletes earlier in the pathway. Interventions like this require adaptation periods, where the ability of technology to monitor performance and allow support like skill acquisition experts to provide feedback is again essential.

Sports, and particularly Para sport, should continue to adopt and adapt with technology and integrate it within their environments where suitable.

Achieving this will allow for improvements in feedback, athlete monitoring, and equipment development. Part of our role as practitioners and researchers is to develop methods to facilitate this and support the development of our coaches and athletes.

References

Abel, T., Burkett, B., Schneider, S., Lindschulten, R., & Strüder, H. K. (2010). The exercise profile of an ultra-long handcycling race: The Styrkeprøven experience. *Spinal Cord, 48*(12), 894–898.

Baumgart, J. K., Brurok, B., & Sandbakk, Ø. (2020). Comparison of peak oxygen uptake between upper-body exercise modes: A systematic literature review and meta-analysis. *Frontiers in Physiology, 11*, 412.

Baumgart, J. K., Gürtler, L., Ettema, G., & Sandbakk, Ø. (2018). Comparison of peak oxygen uptake and exercise efficiency between upper-body poling and arm crank ergometry in trained paraplegic and able-bodied participants. *European Journal of Physiology, 118*(9), 1857–1867.

Buchholz, A. C., & Pencharz, P. B. (2004). Energy expenditure in chronic spinal cord injury. *Current Opinion in Clinical Nutrition and Metabolic Care, 7*(6), 635–639.

Crosland, J., & Boyd, C. C. (2014). Cerebral palsy and acquired brain injuries. In E. Broad (Ed.), *Sports nutrition for Paralympic athletes.* (pp. 91–105). Taylor & Francis Group.

de Groot, S., Bos, F., Koopman, J., Hoekstra, A. E., & Vegter, R. J. K. (2017). Effect of holding a racket on propulsion technique of wheelchair tennis players. *Scandinavian Journal of Medicine and Sport Science, 27*(9), 918–924.

de Groot, S., Hoekstra, S. P., Grandjean Perrenod Comtesse, P., Kouwijzer, I., & Valent, L. J. (2018). Relationships between internal and external handcycle training load in people with spinal cord injury training for the handbikebattle. *Journal of Rehabilitation, 50*(3), 261–268.

De Groot, S., Janssen, T. W., Evers, M., Van der Luijt, P., Nienhuys, K. N., & Dallmeijer, A. J. (2012). Feasibility and reliability of measuring strength, sprint power, and aerobic capacity in athletes and non-athletes with cerebral palsy. *Developmental Medicine and Child Neurology, 54*(7), 647–653.

de Klerk, R., Vegter, R. J. K., Goosey-Tolfrey, V. L., Mason, B. S., Lenton, J. P., Veeger, D., & van der Woude, L. H. V. (2020). Measuring handrim wheelchair propulsion in the lab: A critical analysis of stationary ergometers. *IEEE Reviews in Biomedical Engineering, 13*, 199–211.

Elferink-Gemser, M. T., & Visscher, C. (2012). Who Are the Superstars of Tomorrow? Talent Development in Dutch Soccer. In J. Baker, J. Schorer, & S. Cobley (Eds.), *Talent identification and development in sport: International perspectives* (pp. 99–105). Routledge.

Flueck, J. L. (2020). Body composition in swiss elite wheelchair athletes. *Frontiers in Nutrition, 7*, 1.

Francis, J., Owen, A., & Peters, D. M. (2019). A new reliable performance analysis template for quantifying action variables in elite men's wheelchair basketball. *Frontiers in Physiology, 10*, 16.

Gómez, A. M., Molik, B., Morgulec-Adamowicz, N., & Szyman, R. J. (2015). Performance analysis of elite women's wheelchair basketball players according to team-strength, playing-time and players' classification. *International Journal of Performance Analysis in Sports*, 15(1), 268–283.

Goosey-Tolfrey, V., Keil, M., Brooke-Wavell, K., & de Groot, S. (2016). A comparison of methods for the estimation of body composition in highly trained wheelchair games players. *International Journal of Sports Medicine*, 37(10), 799–806.

Goosey-Tolfrey, V. L., Krempien, J., & Price, M. (2014). Spinal Cord Injuries. In E. Broad (Ed.), *Sports nutrition for Paralympic athletes* (pp. 67–90). Taylor & Francis Group.

Goosey-Tolfrey, V. L., Vegter, R. J. K., Mason, B. S., Paulson, T. A. W., Lenton, J. P., van der Scheer, J. W., & van der Woude, L. H. V. (2018). Sprint performance and propulsion asymmetries on an ergometer in trained high- and low-point wheelchair rugby players. *Scandinavian Journal of Medicine and Science in Sports*, 28(5), 1586–1593.

Janssen, R. J. F., de Groot, S., van der Woude, L. H. V., Houdijk, H., & Vegter, R. J. K. (2021). Towards a standardized and individualized lab-based protocol for wheelchair-specific exercise capacity testing in wheelchair athletes: A scoping review. *American Journal of Physical Medicine and Rehabilitation*. Advance online publication.

Kouwijzer, I., van der Meer, M., & Janssen, T. W. J. (2020). Effects of trunk muscle activation on trunk stability, arm power, blood pressure and performance in wheelchair rugby players with a spinal cord injury. *Journal of Spinal Cord Medicine*. Advance online publication.

Mason, B. S., van der Slikke, R. M. A., Hutchinson, M. J., & Goosey-Tolfrey, V. L. (2020). Division, result and score margin alter the physical and technical performance of elite wheelchair tennis players. *Journal of Sports Science*, 38(8), 937–944.

Mason, B. S., Vegter, R. J. K., Paulson, T. A. W., Morrissey, D., van der Scheer, J. W., & Goosey-Tolfrey, V. L. (2018). Bilateral scapular kinematics, asymmetries and shoulder pain in wheelchair athletes. *Gait Posture*, 65, 151–156.

Mazess, R. B., Barden, H. S., Bisek, J. P., & Hanson, J. (1990). Dual-energy X-ray absorptiometry for total-body and regional bone-mineral and soft-tissue composition. *American Journal of Clinical Nutrition*, 51(6), 1106–1112.

Molik, B., Kosmol, A., Morgulec-Adamowicz, N., Laskin, J. J., Jezior, T., & Patrzalek, M. (2009). Game efficiency of elite female wheelchair basketball players during world championships (gold cup) 2006. *Europenal Journal of Physical Activity*, 22(2), 26–38.

Moore, C. D., Craven, B. C., Thabane, L., Laing, A. C., Frank-Wilson, A. W., Kontulainen, S. A., … Giangregorio, L. M. (2015). Lower-extremity muscle atrophy and fat infiltration after chronic spinal cord injury. *Journal of Musculoskeletal and Neuronal Interactions*, 15(1), 32–41.

Nana, A., Slater, G. J., Stewart, A. D., & Burke, L. M. (2015). Methodology review: Using dual-energy X-ray absorptiometry (DXA) for the assessment of body composition in athletes and active people. *International Journal of Sport Nutrition and Exercise Metabolism*, 25(2), 198–215.

Nevin, J., & Smith, P. M. (2020). The anthropometric, physiological, and strength-related determinants of handcycling 15-km time-trial performance. *Internationl Journal of Sports Physiology and Performance*, 16(2), 259–266.

Rhodes, J. M., Mason, B. S., Perrat, B., Smith, M. J., Malone, L. A., & Goosey-Tolfrey, V. L. (2015). Activity profiles of elite wheelchair rugby players during competition. *International Journal of Sports Physiology and Performance, 10*(3), 318–324.

Richter, W. M., Kwarciak, A. M., Guo, L., & Turner, J. T. (2011). Effects of single-variable biofeedback on wheelchair handrim biomechanics. *Archives of Physical Medicine and Rehabilitation, 92*(4), 572–577.

Rietveld, T., Mason, B. S., Goosey-Tolfrey, V. L., van der Woude, L. H. V., de Groot, S., & Vegter, R. J. K. (2021). Inertial measurement units to estimate drag forces and power output during standardised wheelchair tennis coast-down and sprint tests. *Sports Biomechanics*. Advance online publication.

Simpson, A., Gemming, L., Baker, D., & Braakhuis, A. (2017). Do image-assisted mobile applications improve dietary habits, knowledge, and behaviours in elite athletes? A pilot study. *Sports (Basel), 5*(3), 60.

Sindall, P., Lenton, J. P., Whytock, K., Tolfrey, K., Oyster, M. L., Cooper, R. A., & Goosey-Tolfrey, V. L. (2013). Criterion validity and accuracy of global positioning satellite and data logging devices for wheelchair tennis court movement. *Journal of Spinal Medicine, 36*(4), 383–393.

Stephenson, B. T., Shill, A., Lenton, J., & Goosey-Tolfrey, V. (2020). Physiological correlates to in-race paratriathlon cycling performance. *International Journal of Sports Medicine, 41*(8), 539–544.

Thompson, W. R., & Vanlandewijck, Y. C. (2020). Perspectives on research conducted at the Paralympic Games. *Disability and Rehabilitation, 43*(24), 3503–3514.

Tolerico, M. L., Ding, D., Cooper, R. A., Spaeth, D. M., Fitzgerald, S. G., Cooper, R., ... Boninger, M. L. (2007). Assessing mobility characteristics and activity levels of manual wheelchair users. *Journal of Rehabilitation Research and Development, 44*(4), 561–571.

van der Scheer, J. W., Totosy de Zepetnek, J. O., Blauwet, C., Brooke-Wavell, K., Graham-Paulson, T., Leonard, A. N., ... Goosey-Tolfrey, V. L. (2021). Assessment of body composition in spinal cord injury: A scoping review. *PLoS One, 16*(5), e0251142.

van der Slikke, R. M., Berger, M. A., Bregman, D. J., Lagerberg, A. H., & Veeger, H. E. (2015). Opportunities for measuring wheelchair kinematics in match settings: Reliability of a three inertial sensor configuration. *Journal of Biomechanics, 48*(12), 3398–3405.

van der Slikke, R. M. A., Berger, M. A. M., Bregman, D. J. J., & Veeger, D. (2020). Wearable wheelchair mobility performance measurement in basketball, rugby, and tennis: Lessons for classification and training. *Sensors (Basel), 20*(12), 3518.

van der Slikke, R. M. A., Berger, M. A. M., Bregman, D. J. J., & Veeger, H. E. J. (2016). From big data to rich data: The key features of athlete wheelchair mobility performance. *Journal of Biomechanics, 49*(14), 3340–3346.

van der Woude, L. H., Veeger, H. E., Dallmeijer, A. J., Janssen, T. W., & Rozendaal, L. A. (2001). Biomechanics and physiology in active manual wheelchair propulsion. *Medical Engineering and Physics, 23*(10), 713–733.

Vanlandewijck, Y. C., Evaggelinou, C., Daly, D. J., Verellen, J., Van Houtte, S., Aspeslagh, V., ... Zwakhoven, B. (2004). The relationship between functional potential and field performance in elite female wheelchair basketball players. *Journal of Sports Sciences*, *22*(7), 668–675.

Vegter, R. J., Hartog, J., de Groot, S., Lamoth, C. J., Bekker, M. J., van der Scheer, J. W., ... Veeger, D. H. (2015). Early motor learning changes in upper-limb dynamics and shoulder complex loading during handrim wheelchair propulsion. *Journal of Neuroengineering and Rehabilitation*, *12*(26), 1–14.

12

PHYSIOLOGICAL CONSIDERATIONS FOR PARA ATHLETES

Peta Maloney, Jamie Stanley, Ben Stephenson, and Robert Pritchett
Practitioner Commentary: Gary Brickley

Introduction

An individual's physiological profile is an important factor in their recruitment, classification, and potential for success in Para sport. This chapter will discuss the physiology of common impairments involved in Para sport, and considerations for working with Para athletes to optimise their physiological development. The chapter will finish with two case studies which provide examples of how practitioners have integrated knowledge of physiology with impairment-specific considerations to optimise performance.

Physiology of the main impairments involved in Para sport

Spinal cord injury

The spinal cord has corresponding pairs of spinal nerves exiting the spine at each segment; cervical (C1-C8), thoracic (T1-T12), lumbar (L1-L5) and sacral (S1-S5) (Young, 2021). A spinal cord injury (SCI) to the cervical region is referred to as tetraplegia due to the upper and lower limbs, trunk, and abdomen being affected. A SCI to the thoracic, lumbar, or sacral region is referred to as paraplegia whereby upper limb function remains but the trunk, abdomen and/or lower limbs may be affected (Bhambhani, 2011). Injury to the spinal cord leads to significant motor and sensory deficits and disruption to the autonomic nervous system, with the extent of damage typically greater in an injury higher in the spinal cord. However, a SCI may also be complete or incomplete, the latter leading to some preservation of autonomic function below the SCI level (Roberts et al., 2017).

DOI: 10.4324/9781003184430-12

During exercise, autonomic nervous system dysfunction can reduce physical capacity and performance. Innervation to the sympathetic division of the nervous system exits the spinal cord between T1-T12 (Krassioukov & West, 2014), therefore the extent of dysfunction is dependent on the level of injury. A lack of vasoconstriction and muscle pump activity below the injury leads to impaired blood flow redistribution during exercise (Hopman, 1994). Cardiac output is further reduced in individuals with a SCI >T6 who lack sympathetic innervation to the heart (Krassioukov & West, 2014). Respiratory function is also reduced in individuals with tetraplegia due to the lacking innervation to key respiratory muscles (Haisma et al., 2006). Thermoregulatory capacity may also be compromised due to impaired sweating, shivering, and blood flow responses (Price, 2006).

Despite significant damage to autonomic function arising from a SCI, exercise can improve physiological function. Indeed, trained individuals with a SCI exhibit improved exercise (Hoffman, 1986) and respiratory capacity (Gee et al., 2019) compared to untrained individuals. These adaptations highlight that although the systemic effects of a SCI remain significant, the functional and physiological limitations identified during initial talent identification processes may show some improvement with training.

Limb deficiency

Limb deficiency forms one of the 10 eligible impairments permitted by the International Paralympic Committee for inclusion in Paralympic sports and is defined as '...total or partial absence of bones or joints as a consequence of trauma, illness or congenital limb deficiency' (International Paralympic Committee, 2016, para. 12). Compared to some Paralympic athletes, those with limb deficiency are physiologically more comparable to non-disabled athletes. Nonetheless, pertinent differentiations exist. First, athletes with a lower limb deficiency tend to show greater movement inefficiencies during walking/running (Mengelkoch et al., 2014) and cycling (Elmer & Martin, 2021). These movement inefficiencies raise the energy cost of exercise at a fixed external workload. This effect is greater with ascending levels of impairment (Ward & Meyers, 1995); however, experience and prosthetic advancement may lessen the effect as an athlete transitions into sport (Mengelkoch et al., 2014). Athletes with limb deficiency and their support team should be aware of these inefficiencies to prevent the likelihood of low energy availability (Blauwet et al., 2017) and its associated negative manifestations, or non-functional overreaching (leading to prolonged performance impairment) due to excessive internal training loads (Meeusen et al., 2013). This may be particularly pertinent to developmental athletes who may not be accustomed to the increased energy demands associated with their sport.

Notably, athletes with a limb deficiency display a significant reduction in body surface compared to non-disabled athletes (Webborn & Van de Vliet, 2012). Such an effect reduces the skin surface area available for evaporative heat loss, via sweating, and convective heat loss, via vasodilation of subcutaneous blood vessels; this latter outcome is augmented by narrower arteries proximal to the residual limb (Huonker et al., 2003). The use of prostheses and socket liners further exacerbates the thermal strain imposed on residual limbs by providing an impermeable layer, limiting heat dissipation (Klute et al., 2007) and raising the risk of skin issues (Morris & Jay, 2020). Finally, athletes with an acquired limb deficiency may also possess a considerable area of grafted skin which additionally impairs heat loss (Ganio et al., 2015). Taken together with the aforementioned movement inefficiencies, athletes with a limb deficiency, particularly a lower limb impairment, face a greater thermoregulatory challenge than non-disabled athletes, even more so in hot and/or humid environments.

Neurological impairments

Neurological impairments arise from damage to the central nervous system which may affect physical and/or cognitive performance. This section will cover some of the most common neurological impairments observed in sport, including multiple sclerosis (MS), cerebral palsy (CP) and acquired brain injury.

Multiple sclerosis is a progressive autoimmune disease characterised demyelination of axons of the central nervous system leading to scar formation (Confavreux & Vukusic, 2002). The symptoms that manifest relate to the location within the central nervous system where the scars develop (National MS Society, 2017). Autonomic dysfunction involving gastrointestinal, genitourinary, cardiovascular, and thermoregulatory systems is common (Haensch & Jörg, 2006). Additionally, MS may involve numerous autoimmune cascades, leading to an immune response skewed towards proinflammatory states (Frohman et al., 2006). Given the complex nature of MS, it is unsurprising that many functions critical to sporting performance may be impaired (e.g., balance and skill execution, susceptibility to vibration and peripheral sensory stimulation, and disturbed sleep). Each must be understood in relation to the individual's health and sporting performance requirements, which may also affect the suitability of certain sports during talent identification.

Cerebral palsy is an umbrella term for a group of motor disorders ranging from isolated physical or cognitive impairment to global loss of function (Toldi et al., 2021). It is resultant from an injury to the developing brain during pregnancy or shortly after birth. Muscle control, coordination and tone, reflex, posture, and balance are affected in people with CP with many also having visual, speech, hearing, learning, epilepsy, and intellectual impairments (Vitrikas et al., 2020). Given the diverse clinical presentation of symptoms, impairments to performance may manifest in various ways such as reduced ability to generate power or execute skills, compromised flexibility or range of motion, increased susceptibility to fatigue or seizure risk.

An acquired brain injury occurs when the brain is damaged any time after birth due to accident, illness, stroke or other cause that has long-term effects, and in severe cases can leave people with permanent problems (Healthdirect, 2020). Visual information processing speed may be compromised leading to reduced capacity for decision making, limiting execution of skills, or dizziness among other symptoms (Greenwald et al., 2012). Overstimulation from excessive light and noise may limit ability to perform or execute tasks (Capizzi et al., 2020).

Vision impairment

According to the IPC, athletes with vision impairment 'have reduced or no vision caused by damage to the eye structure, optical nerves or optical pathways, or visual cortex of the brain' (International Paralympic Committee, 2016, para. 18). Similar to athletes with a limb deficiency, those with vision impairment may be considered physiologically comparable to non-disabled athletes. Nonetheless, coaches and practitioners working with these athletes may consider providing greater tactical and verbal feedback during training and competition. Furthermore, typical methods of monitoring hydration through urine colour and volume may be challenging for athletes with a vision impairment (Webborn & Van de Vliet, 2012).

Physiological considerations for working with Para athletes

Physiological testing

Physiological testing provides evidence-based information on an athlete, such as their progress, functional ability and/or areas for improvement. It may also provide valuable insight for talent identification and development purposes, where specific physical and physiological attributes may be particularly desirable for success in certain sports. General principles of physiological testing (Tanner & Gore, 2013) include:

1. Rationale – it is important to have a clear understanding of the purpose of the test, the information collected and how will it be used.
2. Quality assurance – despite testing protocols needing to be modified/ adapted, the credibility and value of results comes from being confident

in the underlying data. The validity of protocols, calibration status of equipment, level of uncertainty in measurement, reporting and documentation protocol modifications must be considered.

3. Standardization – longitudinal monitoring requires data from each lab test to be comparable. Testing equipment, laboratory conditions, nutritional and training status of the athlete should be consistent between testing sessions.

Due to an individual's impairment, adaptations to protocols may/should be considered to ensure the applicability of results. Para athletes are an inherently diverse group and it is highly likely that two athletes with the same impairment will require different testing modifications. Some common considerations are provided below. However, the best source of information regarding necessary modifications/requirements for testing is the athlete themselves. Therefore, prior to any testing, it is important to understand the individual athlete and their specific needs.

Notwithstanding impairment-specific considerations, there are factors ubiquitous to Para athletes that differ from able-body testing guidelines (Stephenson et al., in press).

1. Accompanying carer/handler/nurse present during testing should be acknowledged in any risk assessment.
2. Starting intensities and increments for step or ramp tests should be modified from able-bodied protocols due to impairments and typically shorter training histories.
3. Reference values for physiological parameters (i.e., VO_{2peak}) likely do not exist.
4. Formulae and assumptions for body-composition assessment will be invalid for most Para athletes due to anthropometric differences (Willems et al., 2015).
5. It may not be possible to assess skinfold thickness for each site on the same side of the body. In this instance, a consistent measurement for subsequent tests is required.
6. Due to potential limb deficiencies/impairments in muscle function, it is likely inappropriate to make comparisons between athletes in relative terms (e.g., VO_2 or power output).
7. Venous or arterialized blood sampling using sites on the upper limbs may be challenging due to anthropometric differences (e.g., upper limb deficiencies) or impairments to peripheral blood flow.
8. The maximal rate of oxygen uptake (VO_{2max}) is likely not attained during incremental tests to exhaustion in athletes with impaired muscle function. Therefore, VO_{2peak} is more appropriate.

Training load

Determining training load involves contextualising and synthesising several key training variables, namely duration and intensity, and for decades sport scientists have attempted to quantify these parameters into an encompassing arbitrary metric. Training load is commonly categorised as either internal or external whereby internal training load is defined by the disturbance in homeostasis of the physiological and metabolic processes during the training session (e.g., heart rate) (Borresen & Lambert, 2008). In contrast, external training load is an objective measure of the work that an athlete completes during training (e.g., power output) and is measured independently of the internal workload (Borresen & Lambert, 2008).

Researchers have attempted to quantify training load in a range of Paralympic sports, from Wheelchair Basketball (Iturricastillo et al., 2016) to Para Triathlon (Mujika et al., 2015; Stephenson et al., 2019). Nonetheless, caution should be applied when implementing certain quantification methods in Para athlete cohorts. For example, the commonly used method of calculating a training load value based on athletes' time in pre-determined heart rate zones (Lucia et al., 2003) may be inappropriate for athletes with a SCI above T6. In these athletes, sympathetic denervation limits maximal heart rate to ~120–150 beat·min^{-1}, compressing any submaximal heart rate 'bins' to quantify internal training load (Paulson et al., 2015). Additionally, the use of 'session-RPE' to quantify internal training load may be inappropriate for some athletes. This concept is a simplified approach proposed by Foster et al. whereby a single numerical rating of perceived exertion (RPE) is provided for a training session, using either the 0–10 category ratio or 6–20 scale (Borg & Kaijser, 2006), and multiplied by the session duration (Foster et al., 1995). However, work by Runciman et al. (2015) suggests RPE may be an unreliable measure in athletes with CP, potentially limiting the utility of session-RPE.

Thermoregulation

As previously identified, several Para athletes face unique challenges related to thermoregulation. With the increased globalisation of sports competitions and global warming, athletes will have to contend with challenging environments at all stages of development, not just at the elite level. As such, thermoregulatory capacity may be an important consideration when identifying new athletes. Interventions for athletes with impaired thermoregulation during exercise in hot and humid environments will likely have physiological and psychological benefits. Interventions should be tailored to the individual (Pritchett et al., 2020), based on their impairment, medical history, and training context (see case study). The primary objective is to build athlete confidence that their impairment will not limit their ability to perform via:

- familiarisation to the performance requirements of competition
- development of heat mitigation processes/strategies
- integration of preparation interventions with minimal disturbance to training

Interventions may include heat acclimation, pre-cooling and post-cooling. While elevations in core temperature typically thought to be a prerequisite for heat acclimation (Gibson et al., 2019) may not be attained in all cases, and notwithstanding some equivocal findings for certain impairments (Trbovich et al., 2014), alterations in perceived thermal sensation and sensory responses through peripheral cooling and/or heat acclimation will likely have positive effects on performance. Heat acclimation can be successfully achieved using various modalities including, but not limited to, exercise in the heat (Periard et al., 2015), hot water immersion (Zurawlew et al., 2019), and sauna exposures (Stanley et al., 2015) to stimulate hyperthermia and thermoregulatory adaptation. The physiological benefits from a heat acclimation period (1–2 weeks) can be retained for 4–6 weeks with regular supplemental heat exposures or a shorter re-acclimation block (Saunders et al., 2019). Recent data suggests regular pre-cooling does not attenuate adaptations to training in the heat (Choo et al., 2020). Therefore, for Para athletes who are compromised by sensory responses to heat stress, integration of pre-cooling during an acclimation intervention and pre-competition process may be advantageous (see case study). Recovery from heat stress is critical for adaptations to occur (Daanen et al., 2018), and vitally important for Para athletes susceptible to secondary events such as seizures (Vitrikas et al., 2020), symptom modification and/or fatigue (Davis et al., 2018). Therefore, implementing clear and strategic post-cooling is advised.

Practitioners should adopt a 'minimal effective dose' philosophy when developing solutions to prepare Para athletes for training and competition in hot environments. Cooling interventions implemented pre- or post- acclimation or competition in the heat should consider the event demands and athlete impairments. For example, ice vests and cold-water immersion may have limited feasibility due to logistical challenges in certain situations. Hand cooling, which is cheaper and more portable, and effective in SCI athletes may be impractical due to loss of feeling in the extremities and reduced hand dexterity (Goosey-Tolfrey et al. 2008). Ice slushie consumption is a portable, cost-efficient cooling method that has been shown to be effective at reducing the core temperature when used with cold towels prior to exercise (Forsyth et al. 2016) and expediting the reduction in core temperature following exercise (Stanley et al., 2010). Sometimes the simplest interventions are the most effective and practical, highlighting limited access to resources for developing athletes does not preclude them from implementing appropriate strategies. At the Tokyo 2020 Paralympic Games, commonly used strategies included cold/icy drinks, fans, and damp/iced towels.

Recovery strategies

Recovery from exercise is important for restoring physiological and psychological function. Whilst functional overreaching from training enhances adaptation, the implementation of recovery strategies at targeted times can accelerate recovery time and optimise performance (Kellmann et al., 2018). Commonly used strategies to enhance physiological recovery include sleep, nutrition, hydrotherapy, compression, and massage. The prescription of these strategies should be considered in the context of an individual's needs, as recovery status may depend on several factors including phase of training/competition, nutrition, psychological stress, lifestyle, health, and/ or exposure to environmental stress.

When working with Para athletes, 'impairment' may be another important factor for prescribing recovery due to the physiological consequences of certain impairments. Indeed, Para athletes may be more susceptible to injuries and illnesses (Steffen et al., 2021), highlighting the importance of recovery for optimising health throughout their development. This is particularly important given the reduced pool of individuals that can be recruited into Para sport. Incidental load outside of training may be greater in Para athletes, such as those who compete in a wheelchair who also rely on their upper body musculature for wheelchair propulsion in everyday activities, or those who have an increase in energy cost due to movement inefficiencies (Johnston et al., 2004; Mengelkoch et al., 2014). In addition, sleep is a fundamental recovery strategy (Walsh et al., 2021) yet sleep quality may be worse in athletes with a SCI and athletes with a vision impairment (Tamura et al., 2016). Furthermore, Para athletes with impaired thermoregulation may experience extended post-exercise hyperthermia (Maloney et al., 2021), highlighting the importance of post-exercise cooling. Other physiological consequences such as impaired blood flow may make massage and compression (Vaile et al., 2016) particularly valuable. Massage and stretching also are frequently used as a recovery modality for athletes with increased muscle tone or spasticity. These examples highlight the potentially greater significance of recovery for Para athletes to complement training and optimise adaptation.

Despite extensive research on the effectiveness of various recovery strategies with able-bodied athletes, research with Para athletes is sparse. In the absence of published research and the notable individual differences amongst Para athletes, trialling and refining strategies to suit each individual is critical. Furthermore, Para athletes are often able to provide invaluable experiential input regarding their responses to training and recovery especially in those who have several years of lived experience with their impairment, highlighting the importance of collaboration with the athlete when refining recovery protocols.

Case studies

The following case studies provide examples of physiological monitoring and interventions implemented by practitioners working with Para athletes in applied environments.

Case study 1 – Training load in Para Triathlon

Para Triathlon is a complex multi-modal, multi-impairment endurance sport. As such, it is unsurprising that a single, arbitrary training load metric has not been able to represent the physiological and psychological strain imposed by a training session, microcycle or macrocycle, despite attempts to do so (Mujika et al., 2015; Stephenson et al., 2019), akin to able-bodied triathlon (Cejuela-Anta & Esteve-Lanao, 2011). Instead, it may be more appropriate to visualise training parameters such as volume and intensity distribution separately across the sport's constituent disciplines. In this way, coaches and practitioners can make decisions on athletes' training based upon experience and guided by the basic principles of effective training to aid adaptation and minimise the risk of maladaptation. Below is an example of where this has been applied in practise (Figure 12.1).

Here, the planned and completed weekly/monthly training duration, session-RPE and intensity distribution (using a five-zone model based on physiological testing (Sylta, 2017)) is separated across modalities. From this, rather than using flawed objective guidelines on inappropriate training progressions (e.g., acute/chronic workload ratios; Impellizzeri et al., 2021), athlete support personnel can make decisions with a holistic and con-textualised view for each discipline. Representing completed training re-lative to that which was planned, displaying missed training sessions, is also a key metric given the importance of training availability in individual sports (Raysmith & Drew, 2016), and may highlight unsustainably high training expectations, or overtraining, prior to illness, injury or under-performance. Finally, training intensity may be adapted to suit the intensity distribution model depending upon the aims of the training cycle.

Case Study 2 – Heat preparation of an athlete with Multiple Sclerosis

This case study focuses on the early stage of a Tokyo 2020 Paralympic Games heat strategy for a female athlete with MS consisting of a two-week short-term heat acclimation block. The goal was to familiarise the athlete to

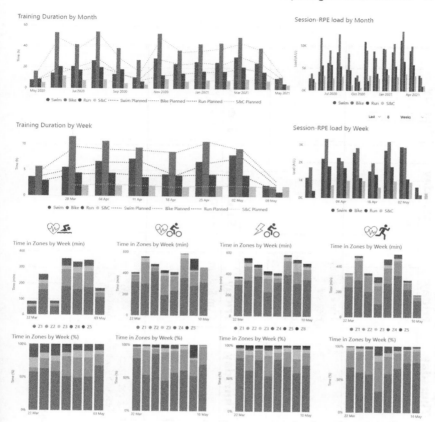

FIGURE 12.1   Example visualisation of training metrics in Para Triathlon

the performance requirements, develop heat mitigation processes, minimising interruptions to training and ultimately to build the athletes' confidence that their impairments would not limit their ability to perform.

The first step was to understand her MS and training history and past experiences with heat stress. Based on this discussion it was identified that she had a previous bad experience with heat stress; she exhibited specific MS-related sensory symptoms in response to heat stress and vibrations from ergometers. Additionally, independent of heat stress, fatigue amplified her MS symptoms. Medical advice indicated that heat stress was unlikely to have long term effects on the progression of her MS. A plan was devised to minimise the risk of these identified negative responses. Part of this plan was to practice cooling processes that would be implemented in Tokyo at the Paralympic Games, including pre- and post-cooling using ice slushies and iced towels with fans for all non-passive heat exposures. The structure of the block is in Figure 12.2.

Monday	Tuesday	Wednesday	Thursday	Friday	Saturday	Sunday
Gym Session	Heat Chamber – Tokyo Specific (27°C, 70% relative humidity)	Recovery ride	Heat Chamber – Aerobic session (35°C, 70% relative humidity)	Gym Session	Rest Day	Endurance ride
Heat Chamber – Heat Stress Test (35°C, 70% relative humidity)		Track session – Heated garments between efforts		Track session – Heated garments between efforts		

Monday	Tuesday	Wednesday	Thursday	Friday	Saturday	Sunday
Gym Session	Heat Chamber – Tokyo Specific (27°C, 70% relative humidity)	Recovery ride		Gym Session	Rest Day	Endurance ride
Recovery ride + Sauna (80°C, 10% relative humidity)		Track session – Heated garments between efforts	Heat Chamber – Heat Stress Test (35°C, 70% relative humidity)	Heat Chamber – Tokyo Specific (27°C, 70% relative humidity)		

FIGURE 12.2 Overview of the two-week heat acclimation block

TABLE 12.1 Specific prescription for the heat stress test session

Step	Duration	Prescription
Step 1	10 min	Power output ~30% anaerobic threshold
Step 2	10 min	Power output ~70% anaerobic threshold
Recovery	5 min	Self-paced recovery
Step 3	15 min	Heart Rate ~75% max
Recovery	5 min	Self-paced recovery
Step 4	15 min	Heart Rate ~75% max

The heat stress test was designed to not only offer a good heat stress stimulus (due to the environmental conditions of 35°C, 70% RH and prescription of workloads – Table 12.1) but provide an assessment on adaptations that have a strong bearing on competition performance.

Based on data from the heat stress test, it was clear that the classic signs of heat acclimation had been achieved (see Figure 12.3) including:

• 7% reduction in HR for a fixed power output
• 45% increased power output for a fixed HR
• 43% quicker duration to reach a core temperature of 37°C (resultant from increased power)
• Delay and reduction in the severity of MS symptoms associated with heat stress
• Increased thermal tolerance evidenced by reduced and delayed perception of thermal sensation, higher sustained core temperature, and mitigation of MS symptoms
• 64% increase in sweat rate

This process instilled confidence in the athlete that heat acclimation and cooling strategies were effective for minimising any negative MS-related symptoms and performance impairment in hot humid conditions. She went on to win a gold and silver at the Tokyo 2020 Paralympic Games.

Concluding remarks

Para athletes possess unique physiological characteristics arising from their impairment. Furthermore, athletes with similar impairment types may respond very differently to the same stimulus. To optimise physiological development, understanding a Para athlete's individual responses in their sporting context is critical. The athlete themselves are an important source of impairment-specific insight, given the variability between Para athletes. To optimise physiological support and performance outcomes, an iterative

(a)

Time point	Tcore (°C)	Tskin (°C)	Power (W)	Cadence (rev.min⁻¹)	Heart Rate (beats.min⁻¹)	Environmental Conditions		Thermal sensation (-5 – +5)	MS Specific scales			
						Temperature (°C)	Relative Humidity (%)		Tingling (1 – 5)	Foot numbness (1 – 5)	Dizziness (1 – 5)	Foot burning/ Stabbing (1 – 5)
Prior to pre-cooling	36.9	31.8										
Step 1 – 10 min	36.0	35.6	78	55	106	35.9	64.8	2.0	1.0	1.0	1.0	1.0
Step 2 – 10 min	36.0	36.9	187	68	148	36.3	67.5	3.0	1.0	1.0	1.0	1.0
Recovery – 5 min	36.2	37.3	63	57	131	36.6	67.5	4.0	2.0	2.0	1.0	1.0
Step 3 – 15 min	36.5	37.3	82	57	128	37.0	67.9	2.7	3.3	3.0	1.0	2.7
Recovery – 5 min	36.8	37.3	29	37	120	37.2	67.7	2.0	2.0	3.0	1.0	4.0
Step 4 – 15 min	37.0	37.5	83	57	128	37.5	66.6	2.0	2.0	2.3	1.0	2.3

	Body mass (kg)	Fluid ingested (kg)	Net weight change (kg)
Pre	64.70	0.70	
Post	64.70		-0.70

(b)

Time point	Tcore (°C)	Tskin (°C)	Power (W)	Cadence (rev.min⁻¹)	Heart Rate (beats.min⁻¹)	Environmental Conditions		Thermal sensation (-5 – +5)	MS Specific scales			
						Temperature (°C)	Relative Humidity (%)		Tingling (1 – 5)	Foot numbness (1 – 5)	Dizziness (1 – 5)	Foot burning/ Stabbing (1 – 5)
Prior to pre-cooling	36.7	24.9										
Step 1 – 10 min	35.1	35.0	80	55	94	35.7	65.8	2.5	1.0	1.0	1.0	1.0
Step 2 – 10 min	35.9	36.0	187	65	138	36.8	61.7	3.0	1.0	1.0	1.0	1.0
Recovery – 5 min	36.6	36.3	62	52	116	35.5	66.5	3.0	1.0	1.0	1.0	1.0
Step 3 – 15 min	36.8	36.1	124	59	128	36.7	64.4	2.3	1.0	1.0	1.0	1.7
Recovery – 5 min	37.1	36.3	58	42	117	36.7	64.8	2.0	1.0	1.0	1.0	3.0
Step 4 – 15 min	37.1	36.3	116	56	129	37.5	64.5	2.3	1.0	1.0	1.0	2.3

	Body mass (kg)	Fluid ingested (kg)	Net weight change (kg)
Pre	63.90	0.95	
Post	63.70		-1.15

FIGURE 12.3 Summary of physiological and perceptual data for the first heat stress test (a) and second heat stress test (b). Data presented are the average for each step. Highlighted cells denote thermal sensations greater or equal to 'hot' and MS-specific scales greater or equal to mid-point between 'no symptoms' and 'worst they've ever been'

process of consulting with the athlete, exploring potential options, and working with the athlete to refine solutions is recommended.

Practitioner commentary

As someone who has worked in Para sport as a physiologist and coach this chapter is valuable for athletes, coaches, academics, students, and anyone contemplating working in sport. The authors have succinctly described physiological development across a range of classifications in Para Sport. There is really good use of up-to-date literature in any area that is ripe for further research. The authors consider a range of impairments, although it is impossible to cover everything in such a brief chapter, they provide the reader a sound appreciation of the physiological demands when working with athletes of various abilities. Although the case studies focus on more endurance-based athletes and preparation in the heat, much of the information is pertinent to other sports. Awareness can help the support staff adapt, reflect, and improve support and performance for the athlete. The SCI section has a greater research emphasis possibly due to more work published in this area and it would certainly be useful to see more on cerebral palsy athletes as this population compete in a range of sports both seated and ambulatory. The day-to-day management of athletes also needs further consideration, but the chapter rightly focuses upon physiological performance.

The case studies provide a useful insight into the training and heat preparation for various events. The balance of training in Triathlon may be needed to meet the development of one athlete's strengths or weaknesses and the individual adaptation to training and equipment should not be underestimated. The perceptual changes in the athlete with MS certainly suggests that the athlete has confidence in the heat acclimation process. The chapter is well referenced which allows readers to explore this area further and consider how they can further their understanding in the field.

References

Bhambhani Y. (2011). *The Paralympic athlete*. Wiley-Blackwell.

Blauwet, C. A., Brook, E. M., Tenforde, A. S., Broad, E., Hu, C. H., & Abdu-Glass, E. (2017). Low energy availability, menstrual dysfunction, and low bone mineral density in individuals with a disability: Implications for the Para athlete population. *Sports Medicine, 47*(9), 1697–1708.

Borg, E., & Kaijser, L. (2006). A comparison between three rating scales for perceived exertion and two different work tests. *Scandinavian Journal of Medicine and Science in Sports, 16*(1), 57–69.

Borresen, J., & Lambert, M. I. (2008). Quantifying training load: A comparison of subjective and objective methods. *International Journal of Sports Physiology and Performance, 3*(1), 16–30.

Capizzi, A., Woo, J., & Verduzco-Gutierrez, M. (2020). Traumatic brain injury: An overview of epidemiology, pathophysiology, and medical management. *Medical Clinics of North America, 104*(2), 213–238.

Cejuela-Anta, R., & Esteve-Lanao, J. (2011). Training load quantification in triathlon. *Journal of Human Sport and Exercise, 6*(2), 218–232.

Choo, H. C., Peiffer, J. J., Pang, J. W. J., Tan, F. H. Y., Aziz, A. R., Ihsan, M., ... Abbiss, C. R. (2020). Effect of regular precooling on adaptation to training in the heat. *European Journal of Applied Physiology, 120*(5), 1143–1154.

Confavreux, C., & Vukusic, S. (2002). Natural history of multiple sclerosis: Implications for counselling and therapy. *Current Opinion in Neurology, 15*(3), 257–266.

Daanen, H. A., Racinais, S., & Périard, J. D. (2018). Heat acclimation decay and re-induction: A systematic review and meta-analysis. *Sports Medicine*, *48*(2), 409–430.

Davis, S. L., Jay, O., & Wilson T. E. (2018). Thermoregulatory dysfunction in multiple sclerosis. *Handbook of Clinical Neurology*, *157*, 701–714.

Elmer, S. J., & Martin, J. C. (2021). Metabolic power and efficiency for an amputee cyclist: Implications for cycling technique. *Journal of Applied Physiology*, *130*(2), 479–484.

Forsyth, P., Pumpa, K., Knight, E., & Miller, J. (2016). Physiological and perceptual effects of precooling in wheelchair basketball athletes. *Journal of Spinal Cord Medicine*, *39*(6), 671–678.

Foster, C., Hector, L. L., Welsh, R., Schrager, M., Green, M. A., & Snyder, A. C. (1995). Effects of specific versus cross-training on running performance. *European Journal of Applied Physiology and Occupational Physiology*, *70*(4), 367–372.

Frohman, E. M., Racke, M. K., & Raine, C. S. (2006). Multiple sclerosis – The plaque and its pathogenesis. *New England Journal of Medicine*, *354*(9), 942–955.

Ganio, M. S., Schlader, Z. J., Pearson, J., Lucas, R. A. I., Gagnon, D., Rivas, E., Kowalske, K. J., & Crandall, C. G. (2015). Nongrafted skin area best predicts exercise core temperature responses in burned humans. *Medicine and Science in Sports and Exercise*, *47*(10), 2224–2232.

Gee, C. M., Williams, A. M., Sheel, W. A., Eves, N. D., & West, C. R. (2019). Respiratory muscle training in athletes with cervical spinal cord injury: Effects on cardiopulmonary function and exercise capacity. *Journal of Physiology*, *597*(14), 3673–3685.

Gibson, O. R., James, C. A., Mee, J. A., Willmott, A. G. B., Turner, G., Hayes, M., & Maxwell, N. S. (2019). Heat alleviation strategies for athletic performance: A review and practitioner guidelines. *Temperature*, *7*(1), 3–36,

Goosey-Tolfrey, V., Swainson, M., Boyd, C., Atkinson, G., & Tolfrey, K. (2008). The effectiveness of hand cooling at reducing exercise-induced hyperthermia and improving distance-race performance in wheelchair and able-bodied athletes. *Journal of Applied Physiology*, *105*(1), 37–43.

Greenwald, B. D., Kapoor, N., & Singh, A. D. (2012). Visual impairments in the first year after traumatic brain injury. *Brain Injury*, *26*(11), 1338–1359.

Haensch, C. A., & Jörg, J. (2006). Autonomic dysfunction in multiple sclerosis. *Journal of Neurology*, *253*(Suppl 1), I3–I9.

Haisma J. A., Van Der Woude L. H. V., Stam H. J., Bergen M. P., Sluis T. A. R., & Bussmann J. B. J. (2006). Physical capacity in wheelchair-dependent persons with a spinal cord injury: A critical review of the literature. *Spinal Cord*, *44*(11), 642–652.

Healthdirect (2020). Acquired brain injury. Retrieved September 28, 2021 from https://www.healthdirect.gov.au/acquired-brain-injury-abi.

Hoffman M. D. (1986). Cardiorespiratory fitness and training in quadriplegics and paraplegics. *Sport Medicine*, *3*(5)312–330.

Hopman M. T. E. (1994). Circulatory responses during arm exercise in individuals with paraplegia. *International Journal of Sports Medicine*, *15*(03), 126–131.

Huonker, M., Schmid, A., Schmidt-Trucksass, A., Grathwohl, D., & Keul, J. (2003). Size and blood flow of central and peripheral arteries in highly trained able-bodied and disabled athletes. *Journal of Applied Physiology*, *95*(2), 685–691.

Impellizzeri, F. M., Woodcock, S., Coutts, A. J., Fanchini, M., McCall, A., & Vigotsky, A. D. (2021). What role do chronic workloads play in the acute to chronic workload ratio? Time to dismiss ACWR and its underlying theory. *Sports Medicine, 51*(3), 581–592.

International Paralympic Committee. (2016). International standard for eligible impairments. Retrieved September 20, 2021 from https://www.paralympic.org/sites/default/files/document/161004145727129_2016_10_04_International_Standard_for_Eligible_Impairments_1.pdf

Iturricastillo, A., Yanci, J., Granados, C., & Goosey-Tolfrey, V. L. (2016). Quantifying wheelchair basketball match load: A comparison of heart rate and perceived exertion methods. *International Journal of Sports Physiology and Performance, 11*(4), 508–514.

Johnston, T. E., Moore, S. E., Quinn, L. T., & Smith, B. T. (2004). Energy cost of walking in children with cerebral palsy: Relation to the Gross Motor Function Classification System. *Developmental Medicine and Child Neurology, 46*(1), 34–38.

Kellmann, M., Bertollo, M., Bosquet, L., Brink, M., Coutts, A. J., Duffield, R., ... & Beckmann, J. (2018). Recovery and performance in sport: Consensus statement. *International Journal of Sports Physiology and Performance, 13*(2), 240–245.

Klute, G. K., Rowe, G. I., Mamishev, a V, & Ledoux, W. R. (2007). The thermal conductivity of prosthetic sockets and liners. *Prosthetics and Orthotics International, 31*(3), 292–299.

Krassioukov A., & West C. (2014). The role of autonomic function on sport performance in athletes with spinal cord injury. *American Academy of Physical Medicine and Rehabilitation, 6*(8), S58–S65.

Lucia, A., Hoyos, J., Santalla, A., Earnest, C. P., & Chicharro, J. L. (2003). Tour de France versus Vuelta a Espa??a: Which is harder? *Medicine and Science in Sports and Exercise, 35*(5), 872–878.

Maloney, P. L., Pumpa, K. L., Miller, J., Thompson, K. G., & Jay, O. (2021). Extended post-exercise hyperthermia in athletes with a spinal cord injury. *Journal of Science and Medicine in Sport, 24*(8), 831–836.

Meeusen, R., Duclos, M., & Foster, C. (2013). Prevention, diagnosis, and treatment of the overtraining syndrome. *Medicine and Science in Sports and Exercise, 45*(1), 186–205.

Mengelkoch, L. J., Kahle, J. T., & Highsmith, M. J. (2014). Energy costs & performance of transtibial amputees & non-amputees during walking & running. *International Journal of Sports Medicine, 35*(14), 1223–1228.

Morris, N. B., & Jay, O. (2020). Aluminium salt-based antiperspirant coated prosthesis liners do not suppress local sweating during moderate intensity exercise in hot and temperate conditions. *Journal of Science and Medicine in Sport, 23*(12), 1128–1133.

Mujika, I., Orbañanos, J., & Salazar, H. (2015). Physiology and training of a world-champion paratriathlete. *International Journal of Sports Physiology and Performance, 10*(7), 927–930.

National MS Society (2017). Symptoms of MS. Retrieved September 27, 2021 from https://www.nationalmssociety.org/Symptoms-Diagnosis/MS-Symptoms

Paulson, T. A., Mason, B. S., Rhodes, J., & Goosey-Tolfrey, V. L. (2015). Individualized internal and external training load relationships in elite wheelchair rugby players. *Frontiers in Physiology, 6*(Dec), 1–7.

Periard, J. D., Racinais, S., & Sawka, M. N. (2015). Adaptations and mechanisms of human heat acclimation: Applications for competitive athletes and sports. *Scandinavian Journal of Medicine and Science in Sports, 25*(Suppl 1), 20–38.

Price M. (2006). Thermoregulation during exercise in individuals with spinal cord injuries. *Sports Medicine, 36*(10), 863–879.

Pritchett, K. L., Broad, E., Scaramella, J., & Baumann, S. (2020). Hydration and cooling strategies for Paralympic athletes: Applied focus: Challenges athletes may face at the upcoming Tokyo Paralympics. *Current Nutrition Reports, 9*(3),137–146.

Raysmith, B. P., & Drew, M. K. (2016). Performance success or failure is influenced by weeks lost to injury and illness in elite Australian track and field athletes: A 5-year prospective study. *Journal of Science and Medicine in Sport, 19*(10), 778–783.

Roberts, T. T., Leonard, G. R., & Cepela, D. J. (2017). Classifications in brief: American spinal injury association (ASIA) impairment scale. *Clinical Orthopaedics and Related Research, 475*(5), 1499–1504.

Runciman, P., Tucker, R., Ferreira, S., Albertus-Kajee, Y., & Derman, W. (2015). Paralympic athletes with cerebral palsy display altered pacing strategies in distance-deceived shuttle running trials. *Scandinavian Journal of Medicine and Science in Sports, 26*(10), 1239–1248.

Saunders, P. U., Garvican-Lewis, L. A., Chapman, R. F., & Periard, J. D. (2019). Special environments: Altitude and heat. *International Journal of Sport Nutrition and Exercise Metabolism, 29*(2), 210–219.

Stanley, J., Halliday, A., D'Auria, S., Buchheit, M., & Leicht, A. (2015). Effect of sauna-based heat acclimation on plasma volume and heart rate variability. *European Journal of Applied Physiology, 115*(4), 785–794.

Stanley, J., Leveritt, M., & Peake, J. M. (2010). Thermoregulatory responses to ice-slush beverage ingestion and exercise in the heat. *European Journal of Applied Physiology, 110*(6), 1163–1173.

Steffen, K., Clarsen, B., Gjelsvik, H., Haugvad, L., Koivisto-Mørk, A., Bahr, R., & Berge, H. M. (2021). Illness and injury among Norwegian Para athletes over five consecutive Paralympic Summer and Winter Games cycles: Prevailing high illness burden on the road from 2012 to 2020. *British Journal of Sports Medicine, 56*, 204–212.

Stephenson, B. T., Hutchinson, M. J., & Goosey-Tolfrey, V. L. (In press). Testing considerations for the ambulant Para-athlete. In *Sport and exercise physiology testing guidelines – Vol 3: Sport testing: The British Association of Sport and Exercise Sciences Guide*. Routledge.

Stephenson, B. T., Hynes, E., Leicht, C. A., Tolfrey, K., & Goosey-Tolfrey, V. L. (2019). Brief report: Training load, salivary immunoglobulin A, and illness incidence in elite paratriathletes. *International Journal of Sports Physiology and Performance, 14*(4), 536–539.

Sylta, Ø. (2017). *Endurance training organization in elite endurance athletes* [PhD thesis, University of Agder]. Research Gate. Retrieved from 10.13140/RG.2.2.1 9966.18240

Tamura, N., Sasai-Sakuma, T., Morita, Y., Okawa, M., Inoue, S., & Inoue, Y. (2016). A nationwide cross-sectional survey of sleep-related problems in Japanese visually impaired patients: Prevalence and association with health-related quality of life. *Journal of Clinical Sleep Medicine, 12*(12), 1659–1667.

Tanner, R. K., & Gore, C. J. (Eds.). (2013). *Physiological tests for elite athletes* (2nd ed.). Human Kinetics.

Toldi, J., Escobar, J., & Brown, A. (2021). Cerebral palsy: Sport and exercise considerations. *Current Sports Medicine Reports, 20*(1), 19–25.

Trbovich, M., Ortega, C., Fredrickson, M. (2014). Effects of cooling vest on core temperature in athletes with and without spinal cord injury. *Topics in Spinal Cord Injury Rehabilitation, 20*(1), 70–80.

Vaile J., Stefanovic B., & Askew C. D. (2016). Effect of lower limb compression on blood flow and performance in elite wheelchair rugby athletes. *Journal of Spinal Cord Medicine, 39*(2), 206–211.

Vitrikas, K., Dalton, H., & Breish, D. (2020). Cerebral palsy: An overview. *American Family Physician, 101*(4), 213–220.

Walsh, N. P., Halson, S. L., Sargent, C., Roach, G. D., Nédélec, M., Gupta, L., ... & Samuels, C. H. (2021). Sleep and the athlete: Narrative review and 2021 expert consensus recommendations. *British Journal of Sports Medicine, 55*(7), 356–368.

Ward, K. H., & Meyers, M. C. (1995). Exercise performance of lower-extremity amputees. *Sports Medicine, 20*(4), 207–214.

Webborn, N., & Van de Vliet, P. (2012). Paralympic medicine. *The Lancet, 380*(9836), 65–71.

Willems, A., Paulson, T. A., Keil, M., Brooke-Wavell, K., & Goosey-Tolfrey, V. L. (2015). Dual-energy X-ray absorptiometry, skinfold thickness, and waist circumference for assessing body composition in ambulant and non-ambulant wheelchair games players. *Frontiers in Physiology, 6*, 356.

Young W. (2021). Spinal cord injury levels and classification. Retrieved September 19, 2021 from https://www.sci-info-pages.com/levels-and-classification/

Zurawlew, M. J., Mee, J. A., & Walsh, N. P. (2019). Post-exercise hot water immersion elicits heat acclimation adaptations that are retained for at least two weeks. *Frontiers in Physiology, 10*, 1080.

13

THE PSYCHOLOGY OF TALENT DEVELOPMENT IN PARALYMPIC SPORT: THE ROLE OF PERSONALITY

Jeffrey J. Martin and Eva Prokesova
Practitioner Commentary: Hannah MacDougall

Personality theory

While limited, research in personality in disability sport has grown in the last 10 years (Martin et al., 2011). For Paralympic athletes, Martin et al., (2011) argued that small effect sizes linked to marginal personality differences may be quite meaningful. For example, Oleksandra Kononova won the 5-kilometer cross-country skiing gold medal at the 2010 Winter Paralympic Games by 2.4 seconds, or the equivalent of .0025% of her time. If remaining relaxed while fatigued, as a function of a personality characteristic like emotional stability, contributes to biomechanical efficiency, it is plausible that a small-time difference of 2.4 seconds may be achievable. Personality traits and PTLID's are different from common sport specific cognitions like wheelchair rugby self-efficacy because they are stable or consistent over time and context (Roberts, 2009). For example, a wheelchair rugby player who is emotionally stable in a sporting context is likely to also be emotionally stable in a work or family context (e.g., parenting upset children). In contrast, that same athlete may have vastly different levels of rugby self-efficacy depending on their recent level of training quality. Personality is also what makes a person unique or distinctive.

In our discussion of personality we emphasize the FFM because of its strong conceptual and measurement underpinnings and history of use for sport-based research (Allen et al., 2011, 2013). The FFM personality constructs are neuroticism, conscientiousness, agreeableness, extraversion, and openness. Neuroticism reflects a person who is frequently anxious and experiences emotional highs and lows. Emotional stability is typically seen as the opposite end of the spectrum from neuroticism in the FFM literature.

DOI: 10.4324/9781003184430-13

Neuroticism is similar to trait anxiety, and in athletics, sport trait anxiety is negatively related to performance, suggesting athletes high in neuroticism will perform more poorly, in general, compared to athletes who are more emotionally stable. Anxious athletes may suffer from less than optimal attentional patterns (e.g., reduced focus) and detrimental changes in motor behavior patterns (e.g., tense muscles) leading to poor performance.

The second factor, conscientiousness, represents individuals who are organized, goal-directed, and detail-oriented which should help athletes engage in high quality and consistent training over time. In particular, such a quality may be particularly helpful for Para sport athletes who often train alone and need to overcome many social-relational (e.g., reduced friendship networks), physiological (e.g., chronic pain), environmental (e.g., inaccessible buses), structural (e.g., no curb cuts), and economic barriers (e.g., underemployment) (Australian Sports Commission, 2011; Casey et al., 2013; Martin, 2012; 2017). Highly conscientious athletes are more likely to develop training plans as well as contingency plans for when training is disrupted (e.g., on holiday, injured). Conscientious athletes are also likely to be diligent about monitoring physiological indices of training and recovery (e.g., resting heart rate) that in turn can be shared with coaches and exercise physiologists.

The third factor is agreeableness. Agreeable athletes are friendly and interested in others. Such qualities should aid team cohesion and coachability. Para sport athletes high in agreeableness may also be well suited to helping novice coaches by being willing to discuss their unique disability specific knowledge and how it influences practice and performance. The fourth factor, extraversion, is not seen as having talent development ramifications to the same degree as the first three FFM dimensions (Kaiseler et al., 2012). However, extraverts have high energy and enjoy being with others suggesting that like agreeableness, team cohesion may benefit from extraverted athletes. The benefits (e.g., social support) of team cohesion may be particularly valuable among Paralympians as they often have to train alone (Caron et al., 2016). Extraversion has also been linked to a problem-focused coping strategies such as increasing effort, seeking out instrumental social support (e.g., teammates to train with) and planning (Kaiseler et al., 2012). The final factor of openness is defined as people who are creative, inquisitive, imaginative, and curious. Although speculative, openness may lead individuals with impairments to try Para sport for the first time. Additionally, openness may help current athletes be more receptive to new training techniques and the many training adaptations that coaches have to make for Para sport. The links from the FFM dimensions to performance, training and talent development, represent the potential direct influence of personality during one specific moment in time. For example, an athlete high in neuroticism may experience anxiety during a critical moment, such as a penalty shot in Para Ice Hockey, which in turn may disrupt concentration, and subsequent performance.

However, many researchers assert that the major influences of personality on performance may in fact be indirect and exert its power over larger time periods (Allen et al., 2011, 2013). For example, personality differences may influence commitment to and quality of practice over a season and even extended periods (e.g., the four years between Paralympic Games). Personality characteristics can also interact. For example, Para sport athletes who are high in extroversion, low in neuroticism, and high in openness used problem-focused coping strategies more so than athletes who do not fit the above profile (Allen et al., 2011). Similarly, Para sport athletes who are high in extroversion, agreeableness, and openness used more emotion-focused coping strategies compared with others. In the following section we discuss personality research conducted with Para sport athletes.

Personality research in Para sport

Sport psychologists often indicate that non-disabled athletes neglect mental skill training. Martin et al. (2011) suggested that this lack of mental skill training is heightened for Paralympians. For instance, Dieffenbach and Statler (2012) reported that 27% of athletes surveyed from the 2010 Winter Paralympic Games indicated that they engaged in no mental preparation prior to the Paralympics. Martin et al. (2011) suggested that the lack of learned mental skills (e.g., relaxation techniques) may make Paralympians more reliant on personality characteristics, such as conscientiousness. Potential Paralympians, as of the writing of this chapter, are training for the Tokyo 2020 Paralympic Games during the Covid-19 pandemic. Preliminary research with 166 Polish athletes training for the Paralympic Games indicates their hours of training were cut in half because of Covid-19 restrictions (e.g., training camps cancelled). Some athletes (12%) stopped training completely and only 5.4% reported having access to sport facilities (Urbański et al., 2021). It is plausible that the training challenges presented by Covid-19 may best be met by athletes characterized as conscientious and emotionally stable (Pété et al. 2021). Understanding how Covid-19 and the ensuing pandemic influenced Paralympic training and post Paralympic performance perceptions is clearly needed.

Martin et al. (2011) compared athletes who made the Paralympic team to those who attended the Paralympics tryout camp but failed to make the team. Athletes making the team went on to win the Paralympic Gold medal. Paralympians were lower in anxiety and higher in tough-mindedness compared to athletes failing to make the team. Recent research on mental toughness has indicated that mentally tough athletes are highly motivated, confident, and focused (Jones et al., 2002; Liew et al., 2019). A personality factor of anxiety reflects the disposition to be tense, worried, and prone to experience emotional highs and lows. Anxious athletes in sport are typically described the same way but their anxiety experiences are specific to sport. Martin et al. (2011) argued that their findings paralleled a large body of research in sport psychology indicating that anxiety usually impairs sport performance. The findings on tough-mindedness, and the questions representing this factor, indicate that athletes who reported they were determined, resolute, and made decisions based on facts and logic (versus intuition) made the Paralympic team, whereas athletes that failed to make the team reported being weaker in these qualities. Finally, as Martin et al. (2011) indicated, the magnitude of personality differences in group membership (i.e., making the team or not) were meaningful as the differences accounted for 25 to 40% of the variance in tough-mindedness and anxiety, respectively.

Personality trait like individual differences (PTLID)

In the next section we focus specifically on three PTLIDs: hardiness, grit, and resilience. Hardiness is defined by feelings of internal control, having a purpose, or meaning in life, and perceiving life difficulties as challenges rather than problems (Martin et al., in press). In non-disabled sport, hardiness is related to success (Golby & Sheard, 2004; Johnsen et. al., 2013), sport engagement (Lonsdale et al., 2007), and subjective well-being (Oliver, 2009). Hardiness is also thought to promote life satisfaction (Pavot & Diener, 1993). Athletes high in hardiness experience satisfaction in their lives because of the three factors constituting hardiness. For example, a person who perceives that her life has a purpose and meaning will more likely feel life satisfaction compared to someone who lacks these life perspectives. Similarly, individuals who feel in control of their life and are aware that their actions and decisions make a difference in their lives, are more likely to feel satisfied than people who lack control. Also being able to view setbacks as opportunities to grow and learn rather than viewing setbacks as difficulties can increase life satisfaction. Hence all three factors constituting hardiness are relevant in promoting behaviors, cognitions, and affect that results in life satisfaction (Martin et al., 2015; Martin et al., 2020).

Grit is defined as perseverance and passion for long-term goals (Duckworth et al., 2007). Researchers have shown that individuals high in grit work hard, maintain their interest and passion despite difficulties and failure, and keep committed to their long-lasting goals (Duckworth et al., 2007; Duckworth et al., 2011). Some authors have suggested that grit promotes life satisfaction because passion is positively correlated to quality of life (Lafrenière et al., 2013). Grit is also positively linked to meaning in life and well-being, resulting in reduced suicide ideation (Kleiman et al.,

2013) and burnout (Salles et al., 2014). It is assumed that athletes high in grit are likely to be satisfied with their lives, because passion and perseverance for their goals provides purpose and direction, which can be a base for increased life satisfaction. It is also thought that athletes high in grit are more likely to be successful in sport, which in turn, can further enhance sport engagement (Atkinson & Martin, 2020; Martin et al., 2015).

Resilience is coping and effectively adapting to trauma, stress, and adversity (Connor & Davidson, 2003), and researchers have revealed its importance in disability contexts (Lindsay & Yantzi, 2014). Resilience is defined more narrowly compared to hardiness and is typically understood as having value when people face adversity, and they have to adjust to major life events (e.g., an acquired impairment) and stressors (Connor & Davidson, 2003). There are various disability-specific challenges that Para sport athletes face in their lives. For instance, some athletes may still be managing emotions (e.g., anxiety, depression) linked to the traumatic event (e.g., car accident) that caused their impairment, health issues connected to their impairment (e.g., pressure sores or chronic pain), or negative social interactions (e.g., discrimination or staring by others: Martin, 2017) that non-disabled athletes typically do not have to face. Previous research in Para sport settings indicates the value of resiliency (Alriksson-Schmidt et al., 2007; Galli & Vealey, 2008). Galli and Vealey (2008) noted that athletes in their study who demonstrated resiliency did so in the face of adversity. Additionally, various psychological strengths (e.g., mental toughness) and social support constituted 'resiliency' and allowed them to manage a plethora of negative emotions (e.g., agitation) and ultimately experience positive outcomes (e.g., motivation to reach out and help others).

Research in personality trait like individual differences

In a series of three studies Martin and colleagues examined how well hardiness, resilience and grit predicted life quality and sport engagement in wheelchair basketball and wheelchair rugby athletes from the USA and the Czech Republic (Atkinson & Martin, 2020; Martin et al., 2015; Martin et al., in press). The following table illustrates the results predicting both life satisfaction and sport engagement (Table 13.1).

The differential pattern of findings involving three different PTLID constructs in predicting life satisfaction and sport engagement indicates that the value of these constructs varies depending on the outcome targeted (Martin et al., 2015). However, in general, it appears that resilience, followed by hardiness and then grit showed the most promise as important PTLID predictors of life satisfaction and sport engagement. It should be noted that grit has recently come under criticism as, to a large degree, it is a

TABLE 13.1 Replication studies of the ability of hardiness, resilience and grit to predict sport engagement and life satisfaction

Citation	Hardiness	Resilience	Grit
Life Satisfaction			
Martin et al. (2015)	.40**	.21*	−.05
Atkinson & Martin (2020)***	.15	.46**	.03
Martin et al. (in press)	.58**	.17	.10
Sport Engagement			
Martin et al. (2015)	.03	.22*	.31*
Atkinson & Martin (2020)***	.27*	.23*	.21*
Martin et al. (in press)	−.17	.43*	.07

*$p<.05$, **$p<.001$.

reformulation of a long-standing personality construct: conscientiousness (Credé et al., 2016). Hence, the modest results in two of the three studies noted above, linking grit to sport engagement in Para sport athletes, can indirectly be seen as supportive of conscientiousness from the FFM.

Personality and PTLID change

Personality is often thought to be stable and enduring, making it somewhat immune to change (Caspi et al., 2005). However recent work generated from a clinical perspective has challenged that view, and to our knowledge this recent work has yet to be embraced by sport psychology researchers (Hudson & Fraley, 2015; Roberts et al., 2017). In a meta-analysis of 207 studies, Roberts and colleagues (2017) found an overall small to medium effect size ($d = .37$) for personality change. In terms of the FFM, the largest to smallest effects were as follows: neuroticism/emotional stability ($d = .37$), extraversion ($d = .23$), conscientiousness ($d = .19$), agreeableness ($d = .15$) and openness ($d = .13$). These findings should be promising for sport psychologists, athletes, and coaches because they suggest that athletes can learn to be more emotionally stable, outgoing, and conscientious. Cognitive behavior therapy, supportive therapy, and psychodynamic therapy were all efficacious in changing personality (Roberts et al., 2017), with the ideal therapy time ranging from four to eight weeks. Interventions lasting less than four weeks saw positive changes drop drastically, and therapy longer than eight weeks only produced marginally larger effect sizes. Optimistically, it was also concluded that changes were robust and lasted at least one year. Roberts et al. (2017) cautioned that the favorable changes may have returned participants to their 'healthy' baseline from a distressed period of their lives. Clearly, generalizing the above results to a healthy population of Para sport athletes should be done tentatively. Finally, behavior, which is so important to sport, was not assessed so the authors could not claim that improvements in emotional stability, for example, produced more adaptive behavior (e.g., an athlete not losing her temper on the court).

Two studies by Hudson and Fraley (2015) addressed the above shortcomings by examining a personality intervention targeting a non-clinical sample and assessing behavior linked to the FFM. They found that participants reported favorable personality changes after a 16-week intervention that used goal setting techniques (e.g., implementation intentions). The findings by Hudson and Fraley (2015) are promising as athletes frequently employ goal setting for physical training (e.g., number of miles to run each week). Coaches, and educational and clinical sport psychologists working with Para sport athletes are also likely to be familiar with many of the effective (e.g., specific) goal setting guidelines advocated by sport psychology researchers. Second, most people want to change their personalities in ways consistent with the FFM (Hudson & Roberts, 2014; Markus & Nurius, 1986) suggesting a lack of motivation will not be a barrier in Para sport settings. For instance, in one study, 97% of the sample wanted to be more conscientious, 89% more agreeable, and 87% more extraverted (Hudson & Roberts, 2014).

Sport psychologists working with Para sport athletes should also be familiar with personality change for another significant reason. Many Para sport athletes were not born with an impairment but acquired one later in life because of a traumatic event (e.g., a car accident). Extreme adverse life events such as a sport (e.g., skiing) or a traffic accident are often associated with changes in personality traits (Lockenhoff et al., 2009). It is not uncommon for athletes who are making their debut at a Paralympic Games to be only a few years post-the traumatic event (Martin, 2017) that caused their impairment, and they may still be making both personality and identity adjustments (Guerrero & Martin, 2018). Adverse life events tend to influence selected facets of neuroticism, openness, and agreeableness. In contrast, extraversion and conscientiousness do not appear to be influenced by extreme life events. Lockenhoff et al. (2009) suggest that the traumatic event leads to anger, hostility, and frustration (elements of neuroticism) and a reluctance to cooperate and deescalate if in conflict with someone else. Finally, they note that their results are similar to how individuals with posttraumatic stress disorder (PTSD) are described. If athletes are preparing for high stake competition such as the Paralympic Games (especially during Covid-19) and managing PTSD or even subclinical PTSD, then sport psychologists and support personal need to be aware of how best to support such athletes which is the focus on the next section (i.e., intervention research).

Applied recommendations

Goal setting

Goal setting is familiar to athletes, and as noted earlier, goal setting for personality change appears to work. More specifically, based on the work of Hudson et al. (2019) goals should be set for behaviors that are consistent with each of the FFM personality traits that athletes may want to change. For example, to develop behaviors consistent with extraversion, an athlete may set a goal of asking a new teammate out for a coffee[1] whereas for conscientiousness, an athlete may start a journal documenting the details of each workout. Similar to the philosophy behind motivational interviewing and performance profiling, athletes should choose (versus being assigned) goals that fit into the FFM. In addition to setting behavior goals consistent with the FFM dimensions, athletes should also employ effective goal setting strategies. For instance, designating the day, time, and where an athlete would ask out a teammate for coffee would fulfill the specificity criteria. Finding a teammate that might have similar goals (e.g., become more extraverted) would provide social support for goal attainment.

Mindfulness

Mindfulness interventions have shown success in non-disabled sport and non-sport disability research for various outcomes, suggesting such interventions may also help Para sport athletes (Gardner & Moore, 2017; Howells & Fitzallen, 2020). Mindfulness often leads to increased self-awareness (Shapiro et al., 2006). When athletes are mindfully aware, they respond to both positive and negative experiences and thoughts in an open and receptive manner. Mindfulness is about freedom from reactivity and habitual reflexive patterns.

Personality change is thought to be a function of many momentary repeated states ingrained into long-term patterns resulting in personality traits. Developing mindfulness may be particularly useful as a vehicle for personality change because it is a reflective process (Wrzus & Roberts, 2017). Reflection allows for time to think about past experiences, feelings, thoughts, and behaviors and relive and reinterpret momentary states. The effects of an eight-week mindfulness intervention for people with spinal cord injuries showed greater improvements in depression, pain catastrophizing, and specific facets (e.g., acting with awareness) of mindfulness compared to those receiving psychoeducation training (Hearn & Finlay, 2018).

Researchers have also examined the effectiveness of mindfulness interventions with non-disabled athletes (Goodman et al., 2014; Gross et al., 2018). Gross et al. (2018) examined the effects of a mindfulness-acceptance-commitment (MAC) intervention compared to traditional PST with female student athletes. Compared to the latter group, athletes in the MAC intervention reported reduced psychological, emotional, and behavioral concerns, and better sport performance. Finally, mindful interventions have helped people with chronic pain (Shapiro et al., 2006). This finding may be particularly important to athletes with impairments as they often experience chronic pain resulting from their impairment (Martin, 2017; Shapiro et al., 2006). In summary, it is plausible to think that similar talent development benefits from mindfulness interventions could be achieved with Para sport athletes. Research determining if mindfulness interventions can help develop talent and how these (better) practices can lead to positive outcomes for related mechanisms (e.g., reduced anxiety) and subsequently, better performances are clearly needed.

Gratitude

> *I think that's key when you're performing because you're in the moment, you're not stressing about the past, you're not stressing about the future, you're just enjoying each and every blessing you have .... So, gratitude gets you in the right state of mind to be able to perform at your best, I believe.*
>
> *(Howells & Fitzallen, 2020, p. 784).*

Gratitude, as the above quote indicates, can influence sport performance. Both state and dispositional gratitude have been shown to enhance psychological, social, and physical well-being (Emmons & Mishra, 2011). Many Paralympians with acquired impairments have faced life-threatening events (e.g., car accidents) that caused these impairments, but have experienced post-traumatic growth (PTG: Hammer et al., 2019). A central feature of experiencing PTG is increased gratitude. In one study of 15 individuals with spinal cord injury (SCI) participants expressed gratitude for everyday life, family support, new opportunities, God, and a positive sense of self (Chun & Lee, 2013). These findings suggest that gratitude linked to impairment is a relevant cognition, suggesting gratitude interventions may resonate with individuals with impairments.

In a study of undergraduate women with trauma history, post-trauma gratitude was positively linked with emotional growth and negatively associated with post-traumatic stress disorder (Vernon et al., 2009). Finally, in a study examining a 90-minute gratitude intervention with college athletes, the participants reported various increases in well-being and decrease in indices of ill-being immediately after and four weeks post-intervention (Gabana et al., 2019). Participants of gratitude interventions have also reported reduced bodily complaints and increased sleep quality (Emmons & McCullough, 2003). Both bodily complaints (e.g., pain) and poor sleep quality (particularly at the Paralympic Games) are problematic for athletes (Rodrigues et al., 2015). Sport psychologists may also consider merging gratitude and mindfulness interventions given they are philosophically compatible. In fact, in one study of student athletes the researchers reported that mindfulness moderated the positive gratitude and life satisfaction relationships. The gratitude and life satisfaction relationship were stronger for athletes high in mindfulness (Chen et al., 2017). In summary, mindfulness and gratitude interventions have shown promise in developing various positive outcomes in non-disabled athletes suggesting they may also be effective in Para sport settings.

Future research directions

We have argued that personality is important, and that personality change is plausible based on prior research and conceptual arguments. However, research specifically with Para sport athletes aimed at talent development is needed. Future researchers should conduct intervention studies examining personality change, related psychological outcomes, and performance using goal setting, mindfulness, and gratitude-based interventions. Longitudinal studies based on the above suggestions would also shed light on talent development in Para sport.

Practitioner commentary

It is clear that both authors have a wealth of understanding and insights into Paralympic sport (and/or adapted sport or sport for all abilities), psychology, mental skills and personality factors. The relevancy of the FFM and PTLID to athletes, coaches, and staff working in Paralympic sport, was firmly established. The authors provided numerous examples and applications of theory and constructs specific for Para sport, thus increasing the relevancy and applicability of the chapter.

Within the chapter, the authors discuss thought-provoking and recent research where data has indicated the potential to change personality, which was previously thought to be relatively constant. It was acknowledged that while this view has yet to be adopted within sport psychology, the authors make insightful applied recommendations based on the view that personality can change over time. The recommendations relating to goal setting, mindfulness and gratitude provide simple and cost-effective ways to potentially improve both athletic performance and the well-being of athletes in Paralympic sports. Moreover, the recommendations are practical in their approach, as well as clearly linked back to FFM and/or PTLID.

Overall, the chapter provides novel and thought-provoking insights into personality and Paralympic sport, however, readers should also consider the wider body of works for topics within the chapter that are not covered in depth (e.g., the concepts of mindfulness and resilience for impact on Paralympic cohorts).

Note

1 Examples are taken from Hudson et al. (2019) and converted to be sport specific.

References

Allen, M. S., Greenlees, I., & Jones, M. (2011). An investigation of the five-factor model of personality and coping behavior in sport. *Journal of Sport Sciences, 29,* 841–850.

Allen, M. S., Greenlees, I., & Jones, M. (2013). Personality in sport: A comprehensive review. *International Review of Sport and Exercise Psychology, 6*(1), 184–208.

Alriksson-Schmidt, A. I., Wallander, J., & Biasini, F. (2007). Quality of life and resilience in adolescents with a mobility disability. *Journal of Pediatric Psychology, 32,* 370–379.

Atkinson, F., & Martin, J. (2020). Gritty, hardy, resilient, and socially supported: A replication study. *Disability and Health Journal, 13*(1), 100839.

Australian Sports Commission (2011). Getting involved with sport: Participation and non-participation of people with disability in sport and active recreation. Sydney, Australian Author, Retrieved on September 30, 2021, from https://www.researchgate.net/publication/235993192_Getting_Involved_in_Sport_The_Participation_and_non-participation_of_people_with_disability_in_sport_and_active_recreation

Caron, J. G., Bloom, G. A., Loughead, T. M., & Hoffmann, M. D. (2016). Paralympic athlete leaders' perceptions of leadership and cohesion. *Journal of Sport Behavior, 39*(3), 219–238

Casey, H., Brady, N., & Guerin, S. (2013). Is seeing perceiving? Exploring issues concerning access to public transport for people with sight loss. *British Journal of Visual Impairment, 31,* 217–227.

Caspi, A., Roberts, B. W., & Shiner, R. L. (2005). Personality development: Stability and change. *Annual Review of Psychology, 56,* 453–484.

Chen, L. H., Wu, C. H., & Chang, J. H. (2017). Gratitude and athletes' life satisfaction: The moderating role of mindfulness. *Journal of Happiness Studies, 18*(4), 1147–1159.

Chun, S., & Lee, Y. (2013). "I am just thankful": The experience of gratitude following traumatic spinal cord injury. *Disability and Rehabilitation, 35*(1), 11–19.

Connor, K. M., & Davidson, J. R. (2003). Development of a new resilience scale: The Connor-Davidson resilience scale (CD-RISC). *Depression and Anxiety, 18,* 76–82.

Credé, M., Tynan, M. C., & Harms, P. D. (2016). Much ado about Grit: A meta-analytic synthesis of the grit literature. *Journal of Personality and Social Psychology, 113*(3), 492–511.

Dieffenbach, K. D., & Statler, T. A. (2012). More similar than different: The psychological environment of Paralympic sport. *Journal of Sport Psychology in Action, 3,* 109–118.

Duckworth, A. L., Kirby, T. A., Tsukayama, E., Berstein, H., & Ericsson, K. A. (2011). Deliberate practice spells success why grittier competitors triumph at the national spelling bee. *Social Psychological and Personality Science, 2,* 174–181.

Duckworth, A. L., Peterson, C., Matthews, M. D., & Kelly, D. R. (2007). Grit: perseverance and passion for long-term goals. *Journal of Personality and Social Psychology, 92,* 1087–1101.

Emmons, R. A., & McCullough, M. E. (2003). Counting blessings versus burdens. *Journal of Personality and Social Psychology, 84*(2), 377–389.

Emmons, R. A., & Mishra, A. (2011). Why gratitude enhances well-being: What we know, what we need to know. *Designing positive psychology: Taking stock and moving forward* (pp. 248–262). Oxford University Press.

Gabana, N. T., Steinfeldt, J., Wong, Y. J., Chung, Y. B., & Svetina, D. (2019). Attitude of gratitude: Exploring the implementation of a gratitude intervention with college athletes. *Journal of Applied Sport Psychology, 31*(3), 273–284.

Galli, N., & Vealey, R. S. (2008). "Bouncing Back" from adversity: Athletes' experiences of resilience. *Sport Psychologist, 22,* 316–335.

Gardner, F. L., & Moore, Z. E. (2017). Mindfulness-based and acceptance-based interventions in sport and performance contexts. *Current Opinion in Psychology, 16,* 180–184.

Golby, J., & Sheard, M. (2004). Mental toughness and hardiness at different levels of rugby league. *Personality and Individual Differences, 37,* 933–942.

Goodman, F. R., Kashdan, T. B., Mallard, T. T., & Schumann, M. (2014). A brief mindfulness and yoga intervention with an entire NCAA Division I athletic team: An initial investigation. *Psychology of Consciousness: Theory, Research, and Practice, 1*(4), 339–345.

Gross, M., Moore, Z. E., Gardner, F. L., Wolanin, A. T., Pess, R., & Marks, D. R. (2018). An empirical examination comparing the mindfulness-acceptance-commitment approach and psychological skills training for the mental health and sport performance of female student athletes. *International Journal of Sport and Exercise Psychology, 16*(4), 431–451.

Guerrero, M., & Martin, J. (2018). Para sport athletic identity from competition to retirement: A brief review and future research directions. *Physical Medicine and Rehabilitation Clinics, 29*(2), 387–396.

Hammer, C., Podlog, L., Wadey, R., Galli, N., Forber-Pratt, A. J., & Newton, M. (2019). From core belief challenge to posttraumatic growth in para sport athletes: Moderated mediation by needs satisfaction and deliberate rumination. *Disability and Rehabilitation, 41*(20), 2403–2411.

Hearn, J. H., & Finlay, K. A. (2018). Internet-delivered mindfulness for people with depression and chronic pain following spinal cord injury: A randomized, controlled feasibility trial. *Spinal Cord, 56*(8), 750–761.

Howells, K., & Fitzallen, N. (2020). Enhancement of gratitude in the context of elite athletes: Outcomes and challenges. *Qualitative Research in Sport, Exercise and Health, 12*(5), 781–798.

Hudson, N. W., Briley, D. A., Chopik, W. J., & Derringer, J. (2019). You have to follow through: Attaining behavioral change goals predicts volitional personality change. *Journal of Personality and Social Psychology, 117*(4), 839–857.

Hudson, N. W., & Fraley, R. C. (2015). Volitional personality trait change: Can people choose to change their personality traits?. *Journal of Personality and Social Psychology, 109*(3), 490–507.

Hudson, N. W., & Roberts, B. W. (2014). Goals to change personality traits: Concurrent links between personality traits, daily behavior, and goals to change oneself. *Journal of Research in Personality, 53*, 68–83.

Johnsen, B. H., Bartone, P., Sandvik, A. M., Gjeldnes, R., Morken, A. M., Hystad, S. W., & Stornæs, A. V. (2013). Psychological hardiness predicts success in a Norwegian armed forces border patrol selection course. *International Journal of Selection and Assessment, 21*, 368–375.

Jones, G., Hanton, S., & Connaughton. D. (2002). What is this thing called mental toughness? An investigation of elite sport performers. *Journal of Applied Sport Psychology, 14*, 205–218.

Kaiseler, M., Polman, R. C. J., & Nicholls, A. R. (2012). Effects of the Big Five personality dimensions on appraisal coping and coping effectiveness in sport. *European Journal of Sport Science, 12*, 62–72.

Kleiman, E. M., Adams, L. M., Kashdan, T. B., & Riskind, J. H. (2013). Gratitude and grit indirectly reduces risk of suicidal ideations by enhancing meaning in life: Evidence for a mediated moderation model. *Journal of Research in Personality, 47*, 539–546.

Lafrenière, M.-A. K., Vallerand, R. J., & Sedikides, C. (2013). On the relation between self enhancement and life satisfaction: The moderating role of passion. *Self and Identity, 12*, 597–609.

Liew, G. C., Kuan, G., Chin, N. S., & Hashim, H. A. (2019). Mental toughness in sport. *German Journal of Exercise and Sport Research, 49*(4), 381–394.

Lindsay, S., & Yantzi, N. (2014). Weather, disability, vulnerability, and resilience: Exploring how youth with physical disabilities experience winter. *Disability and Rehabilitation, 36*, 2195–2204.

Lockenhoff, C. E., Terracciano, A., Patriciu, N. S., Eaton, W. W., & Costa Jr., P. T. (2009). Self-reported extremely adverse life events and longitudinal changes in five-factor model personality traits in an urban sample. *Journal of Traumatic Stress, 22*, 53–59.

Lonsdale, C., Hodge, K., & Jackson, S. A. (2007). Athlete engagement: Development and initial validation of the Athlete Engagement Questionnaire. *International Journal of Sport Psychology, 38*, 471–492.

Markus, H., & Nurius, P. (1986). Possible selves. *American Psychologist, 41*(9), 954–969.

Martin, J. (2019). Is the profession of sport psychology an illusion? *Kinesiology Review, 9*(2), 92–103.

Martin, J. (2012). Mental preparation for the 2014 Winter Paralympic games. *Clinical Journal of Sport Medicine, 22*(1), 70–73.

Martin, J. J. (2017). *Handbook of disability sport and exercise psychology.* New York, NY: Oxford University Press.

Martin, J. J., Byrd, B., Watts, M. L., & Dent, M. (2015). Gritty, hardy, and re-silient: Predictors of sport engagement and life satisfaction in wheelchair basketball players. *Journal of Clinical Sport Psychology, 9*, 345–359.

Martin, J. J., Dadova, K., Jiskrova, M., & Snapp, E. (in press). Sport engagement and life satisfaction in Czech parasport athletes. *International Journal of Sport Psychology.*

Martin, J. J., Malone, L. A., & Hilyer, J. C. (2011). Personality and mood in women's Paralympic basketball champions. *Journal of Clinical Sport Psychology, 5,* 197–210.

Oliver, C. M. (2009). Hardiness, well-being, and health: A meta-analytic summary of three decades of research (Doctoral dissertation). Available from ProQuest Dissertations and Theses database (UMI No. 3391674).

Pavot, W., & Diener, E. (1993). Review of the satisfaction with life Scale. *Psychological Assessment, 5*(2), 164–172.

Pété, E., Leprince, C., Lienhart, N., & Doron, J. (2021). Dealing with the impact of the COVID-19 outbreak: Are some athletes' coping profiles more adaptive than others?. *European Journal of Sport Science, 22*(2), 1–27.

Roberts, B. W. (2009). Back to the future: Personality and assessment and personality development. *Journal of Research in Personality, 43,* 137–145.

Roberts, B. W., Luo, J., Briley, D. A., Chow, P. I., Su, R., & Hill, P. L. (2017). A systematic review of personality trait change through intervention. *Psychological Bulletin, 143*(2), 117–142.

Rodrigues, D. F., Silva, A., Rosa, J. P. P., Ruiz, F. S., Veríssimo, A. W., Winckler, C., … & de Mello, M. T. (2015). Sleep quality and psychobiological aspects of Brazilian Paralympic athletes in the London 2012 pre-Paralympics period. *Motriz: Revista de Educação Física, 21*(2), 168–176.

Salles, A., Cohen, G. L., & Mueller, C. M. (2014). The relationship between grit and resident well-being. *American Journal of Surgery, 207,* 251–254.

Shapiro, S. L., Carlson, L. E., Astin, J. A., & Freedman, B. (2006). Mechanisms of mindfulness. *Journal of Clinical Psychology, 62*(3), 373–386.

Urbański, P., Szeliga, Ł., & Tasiemski, T. (2021). Impact of COVID-19 pandemic on athletes with disabilities preparing for the Paralympic Games in Tokyo. *Research Square, 14*(1), 233.

Vernon, L. L., Dillon, J. M., & Steiner, A. R. (2009). Proactive coping, gratitude, and posttraumatic stress disorder in college women. *Anxiety, Stress, and Coping, 22*(1), 117–127.

Wrzus, C., & Roberts, B. W. (2017). Processes of personality development in adulthood: The TESSERA framework. *Personality and Social Psychology Review, 21*(3), 253–277.

14

THE OVEREMPHASIS ON 'TALENT' IN PARA SPORT DEVELOPMENT

P. David Howe and Carla Filomena Silva
Practitioner Commentary: Raphael Moreira de Almeida

It takes a tremendous amount of time, effort, and money to train an athlete from the stages of developmental physical literacy that often initially occurs within the family and physical education classes at school to the elevated position at the top of an Olympic Games podium. The time, commitment, and effort on the part of the athlete and close family members, friends, and numerous coaches as the athlete develops is immeasurable. Factoring in support from local, provincial, and national sports organisations also adds to the task of quantifying the cost of talent development. It takes years and years of hard work to produce an Olympic champion. In the case of Paralympic sport, the route for developing a champion is often not as long or as unpredictable for a number of reasons. For instance, people who experience disability are less likely to be physically active in comparison to those who are considered able because of multiple impediments to participation (Rimmer & Marques, 2012). Related to this, not many individuals who possess Paralympic eligible bodies are physically active globally (Office of the UN High Commissioner for Human Rights, 2021).

The classification process is much more complex in Paralympic sport than in its mainstream counterpart. Bodies are not simply classified by sex and weight categories, instead Paralympic sport classification is a process whereby athlete's bodies are put through a number of functional and/or medical evaluations to determine whether they are eligible to compete in events governed by the International Paralympic Committee (IPC) (Howe & Jones, 2006; Howe 2008a). Because of the complexity of the system and the IPC's desire to level the playing field for a diverse population who experience disability within Paralympic sport, there are multiple competitive classes for both men and women at the Paralympic Games. Due to the

DOI: 10.4324/9781003184430-14

fewer bodies eligible to compete in a variety of classes, reaching the podium in Paralympic sport becomes numerically easier. Thus, predetermining who has better chances to be a successful Paralympian is not as uncertain as it is within the Olympic realm, but it is still a complex process, dependent upon a multitude of factors such a type and severity of impairment, and body phenotype for example have an impact upon talent (see Chapter 6 for more on Paralympic classification systems).

The identification of talented individuals within society is not a new pursuit. It is something that has interested pedagogues, coaches, and talent agents from a variety of fields for centuries. How to nurture and develop our progeny has long fascinated us and central to these discussions has been a focus on the 'nature vs nurture' debate (see Baker & Young, 2020) and the facilitation of an environment in which 'natural' talents can germinate. Writing in the middle of the last century, Faris suggested:

> A major difficulty in the study of environmental causes of genius has been the formulation of an adequate conception of environment. In order to arrive at such a definition it is necessary to determine what factors in the experiences and surroundings of persons studied might have produced their abilities.
>
> *(Faris, 1936, p. 538)*

In other words, the determinants of elite performance exist at the intersection of individual talent (both innate 'fixed' individual qualities and developed traits and skills), other individual characteristics (age, physical qualities, early experiences and stimulus in particularly critical periods for motor development), the quality of training practices and other environmental factors (e.g., practical conditions to access high quality training) (Ackerman, 2014). But we cannot move forward without a robust understanding of what individual talent entails, and once again, we refuse the extremes of nature (innate and fixed qualities) versus nurture (environmental input) position. We anchor our analysis in Ackerman's definition of talent as:

> the individual's current standing on various dimensions of individual differences (e.g., cognitive, affective, conative). These traits arise through a complex interaction of genetics and environment, but once developed, are relatively stable and important determinants of future behaviors and skill development.
>
> *(2014, p. 12)*

The belief that talent, as an innate quality does not exist, but can instead be grown has also become a hallmark concept within the non-fiction popular publishing surrounding the concept (Colvin, 2010; Coyle, 2009; Gladwell, 2008). Middle class parents have long dialled into this view that talent is a product of meritocracy, but recent research has burst this bubble (Littler, 2018). The meritocracy narrative is as old as the beginnings of modern sport, when middle-class men exceled because the structure and organisation of these developing forms of leisure (and sport) required time (more than talent) – something that working men[1] did not have in abundance (Gruneau, 1999; Hughson, 2009). Within the context of sport there has been an increased attention paid to the talent identification and development and the tensions therein (Baker et al. 2017, 2018, 2020), as well as specifically within the context of Paralympic sport (Dehghansai et al., 2020, 2021). Ultimately, such work highlights that *talent searches* for medallists are not only complex and multifactorial, but also have limited utility.

So where does this leave us with regards to debates surrounding talent development in Paralympic sport? The authors of this chapter have a wealth of experience within Paralympic sport that inform the (perhaps unpopular) argument that follows. With a lifetime of experience of disability including time as an athlete and advocate within Paralympic sport (see Howe, 2018), the first author draws upon a distinctive understanding of the Paralympic sport practice community (Howe & Jones, 2006). The second author has extensive ethnographic experience within the development of sitting volleyball (Silva, 2013; Silva & Howe, 2019) which is vital in our understanding of this issue. Together, their experiences within individual and team sport practice communities (Morgan, 1994) will be useful to elucidate our views of the importance of fast-tracking talent identification.

While debates regarding what is talent and how can it be developed are interesting and have been the focus of much high-quality research (Baker, et al. 2017, 2018, 2020) in this chapter we are questioning the utility of Paralympic sport talent identification events and talent transfer programs. We feel these programs run counter to the development of a sustainable and inclusive Paralympic sport movement. To illuminate our argument, we will highlight how the shift from Paralympic sport for participation to high-performance has had a detrimental impact on the numbers of athletes competing, especially athletes seen as more severely disabled (Howe, 2008b). The acceleration of 'professional' Paralympic sport, with most of the leading western nations paying athletes also has had negative consequences on the development of grassroots sports in many countries. Related to this is the obsessive pursuit of medals, seen as the hallmark of a successful National Paralympic Committee (NPC) (Radtke & Doll-Tepper, 2014). The quest for medals leads nations to shortcut the development of Paralympic programs, in particular through talent transfer initiatives. We will argue that these developments, which are a product of the neoliberalisation of sport (Andrews &

Silk, 2018) run counter to the International Paralympic Committees (IPC) mission to be a vanguard for inclusion in sport.

We start our examination by providing a brief background of the Paralympic movement before turning our attention toward the task of finding and developing Paralympic sport talent in contemporary contexts. Our attention then shifts to the value of talent transfer within Paralympic sport and we close the chapter by discussing the whole process of talent identification and the impact that it can have upon the Paralympic sport practice community (Morgan, 1994; Howe & Jones, 2006).

Historical background

Disability sport, as the foundation for the Paralympic Movement was used as a vehicle to enhance the rehabilitation of British ex-servicemen during the second world war (see Chapter 2 for a brief overview of the Paralympic evolution, Guttmann, 1976). These individuals were not simply doing sport for the sake of it, but rather to become employed members of society and ultimately taxpayers (Anderson, 2003). Early on, such sporting opportunities were only available for individuals who suffered from spinal cord injuries, though the Paralympic sport movement did expand to include individuals with other impairments prior to the 1980s (Howe, 2008b). The desire to re-habilitate injured bodies by using sport is still seen today, as people who experience disability are often directed to participate in sport as part of their rehabilitation process (Seymour, 1998). The rationale is that getting involved in a grassroots sports program will aid their rehabilitation by enhancing bodily movement and providing a social outlet into the broader community.

As more athletes shifted from rehabilitation to participation in the context of what Guttmann (1976) termed *sport for the disabled,* opportunities to compete internationally developed. As a result, a number of International Organisations of Sport for the Disabled (IOSD) were formed to enable athletes from around the world to compete in sport on a level playing field. These organisations were structured around particular impairment groups (spinal cord injuries – where individuals were often confined[2] to a wheelchair, visually impaired, hearing impaired[3], cerebral palsy, and amputees). The IOSDs introduced systems that were designed to create a level playing field by establishing distinctive classification systems for each impairment group (Howe & Jones, 2006). As more athletes began to compete internationally, there was a push to focus upon *high-performance* Paralympic sport which ultimately led to the establishment of the International Paralympic Committee (IPC) in Dusseldorf on September 21, 1989 and officially began the Paralympic Movement (Howe, 2008b).

This brief history of the Paralympic movement and its three related stages (rehabilitation, participation, and high-performance) is essential to consider when debating the importance of talent within Paralympic sport. The focus on both rehabilitation and participation aims at the individual's development. Rehabilitation allows individuals to develop skills that will help in their reintegration into society. Whether this means undergoing remedial training through physical or occupational therapy, facilitating independent living for someone who has a congenital impairment, or the process of re-embodiment following traumatic injury (Seymour, 1998), the foundational principle behind rehabilitation is to enhance an individual's quality of life and social inclusion. There is also a belief that participation in sport can enhance quality of life, but doubts remain as to whether high-performance Paralympic sport can do the same (Howe & Silva, 2018; Silva & Howe, 2018).

Finding and developing Para sport athletes: Teams versus individuals

The identification of potential successful Paralympic sport athletes within western sports systems often relies upon talent searches relying upon physical attributes validated through physiological testing (Baker et al., 2020). Both authors of the chapter have attended numerous talent identification events organized under the umbrella of 'Paralympic development'. Our experiences left us with concerns for the well-being of athletes, both those identified as 'talented', but, perhaps more importantly, for those who were not. The nature of formal talent identification programs left us also concerned about the long-term sustainability of Paralympic sport as a vehicle to enhance participation in sport for all individuals who experience disability. Our experience of these days varied in part because of the nature of the sport which was the focus of talent identification. In other words, there are different expectations for talent identification within the team and individual sports.

Team talent identification

When a Paralympic sport organisation wants to recruit team players to a program the pressure to identify enough players overrides the search for 'talent'. For instance, players may be successful in being recruited simply because their physicality fits the need of the sport. If a program is in its developmental stage, managers may be looking simply for bodies with the *right* impairment. For example, in sitting volleyball double above the knee amputees are often considered ideal (Silva, 2013), because the lower limb gets in the way when moving around the court. In scenarios like this, there is potential for the new developing program to keep athletes involved in the program (often at their own expense) who have no previous experience or special talent for the game – simply because the national federation needs a certain number of players for the program to be considered worthy of funding (Silva, 2013).

If the talent identification event is held for an established program (that has represented the nation at previous Paralympic Games), the recruitment of new players often happens at training camps where established national team athletes compete for a place against invited players from outside the squad who have a desire and the presumed talent to play the sport at the elite level. The coaches and staff of the program in a training camp environment are trying to find 'new blood' that will enhance the team's talent and opportunity to get to the podium. Seldom does this kind of talent identification process trigger a big programmatic shift, unless a new coach or management team has just been appointed. However, when the team in question has little or no Paralympic pedigree and is trying to establish itself – athletes are more prone to be used as means to someone else's agenda, namely the managers', national sport organizations' or the NPC's.

In establishing a team program, athletes need to be willing and able to train with the team – even if selection for the Paralympic Games is not yet guaranteed. Some players have been known to have been strung along in these contexts with no realistic chance of being part of the Paralympic program (Silva, 2013). While the athlete's body may be eligible for the particular sport, they may lack the required skill level to excel at the international stage. As some sport programs struggle to gather enough athletes, their chances of receiving funding from central funding bodies are also compromised, and so the pressure to recruit and potentially exploit eligible players, regardless of their 'talent'. Their body is of value – just not on the field of play.

Individual sports

Talent identification days for individual sport are different to team sports because the outcome does not rely upon having enough eligibly impaired bodies. Rather, coaches are looking for a 'golden needle' in a haystack (Dehghansai et al., 2021). As such, athletes attending the Paralympic sport talent identification event are more likely to be driven by the dream of becoming a Paralympian because this is dependent directly upon their body rather than the collective ability of teammates.

Individual sport programs at talent search events go about finding athletes that meet their physical requirements by putting them through a battery of physiological tests to assess how their bodies measure up on key performance indicators. Thus, despite talent being multifactorial–the performance at a one-off event can determine the athlete's sporting fate. Despite a large number of athletes attending these events, because the goal of these events is to sign up potential medallists, there is often no follow-up if their body is seen as irrelevant to join the elite quarters of the NPC program. This is a huge, missed opportunity to grow grassroot Paralympic sport provision and is ethically problematic. While recent talent identification research conducted with so-called Paralympic sport experts (Dehghansai et al., 2021) highlights they need to know more about impairments and classification, one is left wondering what distinctive knowledge is needed to validate talent ID programs in Paralympic sport? What distinguishes Paralympic sport from non-disabled sport is the knowledge of the intersections between classification systems, impairment, disability, and performance (Howe, 2008a, 2008b). One assumes in this research, the term *expert* was used because individuals worked within the Australian Paralympic sport system, but like the ambiguous concept of talent, within this field, what constitutes expertise and expert knowledge needs to be further scrutinised. Until this is done, the already weak foundations of talent identification programs will be further undermined. Before robust talent ID processes can be designed, we need to know more about the dynamic of the intersection between impairment, disability, performance, and talent; and how Paralympic talent can be fostered, rather than assuming it can be 'found'.

Talent transfer: 'Robbing Peter to pay Paul'

We have briefly discussed talent searches as a tool to enhance the identification of potential international medallists as they relate to the broad distinction between team and individual sports. There is however another common, yet problematic practice, the talent transfer system. This system entails that once athletes have been recruited to national programs, they may become 'wanted' by other sports federations as part of the talent transfer system. A talent transfer system might benefit someone who wishes to continue at a high level in sport but is not effective at sustaining world leading performances any longer within the sport where they entered the elite sport system. In Canada, for example, 'the Canadian Paralympic Committee (CPC) began a new initiative – Paralympian Search – which is held across Canada, three or four times a year, with the purpose of increasing awareness, attracting novice athletes, and providing opportunities for experienced athletes to transfer between sports' (Dehghansai & Baker, 2020, p.130). Such programs cover both the talent search and transfer because of the small number of athletes involved – 225 over a 2-year period (Dehghansai & Baker, 2020, p. 129).

Within the Paralympic sport program over the last decade, there have been several new Paralympic eligible sports that have unceremoniously and illicitly recruited athletes established in other sports, with the lure of improved financial support and the opportunity to gain Paralympic selection, which may have passed them by in their chosen sport. Talent transfers can fast track athletes towards medals, particularly in new Paralympic sports programs which may have no grassroots sporting development strategy. The 'transferred' athletes may find their move financially rewarding, but they often struggle because the culture within the practice community of the new Paralympic sport may be only tangentially related to the sport that was their first love (Howe & Jones, 2006). Initially, athletes are drawn to a particular sporting practice because of the internal goods, with this intrinsic motivation being paramount to the quality and longevity of their commitment to a community of like-motivated individuals, united by the valuing of similar internal goods accrued from practising the sport (Morgan, 1994). These internal good are constitutive of the distinctive sporting communities. In fact,

> The concept of "internal goods" is crucial in our analysis because they are distinctive to the practice in question. They are partly definitive of the practice, and their achievement provides the motivation for participating in "this" practice rather than "that" one. Internal goods are peculiar to a particular practice and cannot be achieved in any other way save participation in that practice.
>
> *(Howe & Jones, 2006, p. 33)*

Therefore, this understanding of engagement in a sport as grounded in a community of practice is significant because of how an athlete's relationship with the practice can enrich them as individuals and become so central to their identities (Howe & Jones, 2006). For example, transferring from running track to rowing implies a much different community of practice, a distinctive sporting culture grounded in different core values and internal goods. The 'transferred' athletes overlook these distinctions, as they are, often, distracted or solely motivated by the external goods (such as money, medals, and sponsorship) obtained by the minority, which compromises the long-term sustainability of the whole sporting practice community (Morgan, 1994).

Of course, organisations at the heart of talent transfer systems such as NPCs are vocal about the health and well being of the transferring athletes (Dehghansai, 2021) but such rhetoric while good for the public image, is seldom the real priority of a high-performance sports organisation, pressured by the need to show 'tangible' success. Sporting organisations are judged and funded by the medals won, and therefore should not be judged poorly because they engage in such rhetoric and ethically questionable practices such as the talent transfer programs. Rather, critical thinkers should be mindful that the agenda of an NPC, in the context of professional Paralympic sport is governed by a neoliberal agenda: to enhance national pride (and accrue the correspondent financial rewards) by climbing the medal table. This is why NPCs are supported by their governments. Talent transfer programs that fast-track athletes from one high-performance system to another where grassroots development is non-existent are designed to enhance sporting programs access to the external rewards to the detriment of long-term sustainable development.

Discussion

A systematic review of talent identification and sport conducted by Johnston et al. (2018) highlights a lack of consensus in the literature between the skill levels athletes require to be successful. This suggests to us as social scientists that determining talent, recruited to high-performance pathways or transferred between competing sport is nowhere near an exact science. Clearly, there is a lack of clarity regarding what makes an athlete a winner. We may start to ask ourselves 'What is the point of talent identification, then?' If it is so difficult to define what talent is, even considering sport specific physical prowess and the biomechanical and physiological parameters, then engaging in the pursuit of fast-tracking talent identification is at best, irrelevant, at worst, harmful.

Massey and Whitley (2021) have nicely articulated the concept of the talent paradox in the context of elite youth sport. While not the same as Paralympic sport, this concept can be utilised while critically exploring the world at the heart of this chapter. Massey and Whitley (2021) highlight that while elite sporting programs can be filled with rewards (the external good highlighted above) they can just as easily be filled with disillusionment, disengagement, and damage. In other words, 'success at the elite youth level often forces athletes to walk a 'tight rope' in which talent progression and winning are predicated on sacrificing holistic development and well-being' (Massey & Whitley, 2021, p.167). Programs for talent identification and transfer may lead nations to a more elevated status on the medal table, but at what cost to long-term athlete development and health and well-being?

Conclusion

It is important the readers realise; in this chapter we are not arguing that NPCs are acting inappropriately – they are caught in the neo-liberal market where their funding is predicated on producing golden moments of national pride for the tax paying public. Goals of long terms sustainable high-quality sports programming in practice fall outside their remit. Finding and harnessing talent today is seen as the hallmark of a successful NPC and a nation in terms of opportunities provided for people who experience disability. Those that achieve success every two years as celebrated through the summer and winter Paralympic medal table will be handsomely rewarded for this. But what of the long-term development of Paralympic sport participation?

Attempts to codify talent and its identification and transfer between practice communities are a product of neoliberalism and run counter to ideas of participation development. They have negative consequences upon grassroot development as organisations are not rewarded for slow and methodical sustainability. Yet we believe they should be. The internal goods of a sporting practice community are far more relevant to the betterment of the human condition than a golden shower of medals every two years.

Whether the body that joins the Paralympic sport practice community is talented should be immaterial to the enjoyment of the endeavour.

> Often a very trivial experience will set off a chain of results that affects the entire character of the person. The unique sequence of events, and interrelations of personality, social background, opportunities, relations with members of the family and other groups, while necessarily different for each person, must enter into the explanation of the development of abilities
>
> *(Faris, 1936, p. 544)*.

In other words, developing practice communities of sport that share experiences and positive values while engaging in worthwhile physical and social development should be our end game.

Practitioner commentary

In my country, Brazil, the government invests millions of reais per year to finance Para sport and all the structures athletes need to achieve impressive results and medals in world competitions. Since the Beijing 2008 Paralympic Games, Brazil is in the top 10 of the medals table, being part of an elite Paralympic Movement. Talent identification and development is an important part of those investments, with a special space for the Scholar Paralympics (Paralimpíadas Escolares in Portuguese), which is the biggest event for people with impairments at school ages. In 2019, 1,200 athletes were part of this program, which has already revealed Paralympic medalists Alan Fonteles (Para Athletics), Petrúcio Ferreira (Para Athletics) and Bruna Alexandre (Para Table Tennis).

Our country's results were improving in the Tokyo 2020 Paralympic Games, we had the best result in our history, with 72 medals in total in the 7th position in the medals table. The expectations for the future look bright, as we also have one of the best Para Training Centers in the world, in São Paulo. While Brazil has demonstrated its Paralympic power, is this development and growth sustainable? Will the sport be accessible for all people with impairments in the country despite earning so many laurels at the Paralympic Games? According to my experiences, unfortunately, no.

During my nine-year tenure in Para sport, I have worked within high-performance and participation programs. For the fortunate athletes that are identified as potential medallists and future 'Para stars', Brazil (National Paralympic Committee and national federations) ensure all their needs are met (i.e., training facilities, coaches, sponsorship, and international competitions). But unfortunately for the other 'less talented' athletes, or even people with impairments that have never practiced any sports, we don't have facilities to allow them to be active and participate in Para sport.

In my first job, I had around 18 children and teenagers with impairments learning Para table tennis – PTT. After one year, the company that sponsored the project stopped their investments and we were forced to stop our activities. The biggest problem was that, from one day to another I didn't have any solution for them to continue practicing the sport, because we did not have a lot of specialized clubs for Para sport in Brazil, and even less for PTT. Fast forward several years and only one of my students from that time still plays PTT. What if the other participants had more opportunities to continue? In hindsight, if the program had continued, we had more chances to have more talents developed in PTT; while my students would still be physically active, even if they had no intention to follow the high-performance path.

That is why this chapter is so important for your understanding of talent identification and development, dear reader. The authors show to us how talent ID is being done and how it should be: with long-term sustainable Para sport programs, which offer opportunities to practice to all people with impairments, and not only for some of the 'most talented' of the bunch. In this way, we can discover and develop Paralympic medallists, but we also give opportunities to those who want to practice for other reasons including health and enjoyment. So, we will include, not exclude.

Notes

1 The development of sport as we know it today was targeted at men. For working men it was considered an opiate for the masses – designed to distract them from their poor quality of life (see Brohm, 1989). For the middle classes sport was designed to distinguish them from the working classes and was an amateur pursuit where leisure time was required (Sheard & Dunning, 1979).

2 The use of the word 'confined' is purposeful here, as this was the rhetoric that would have been seen as appropriate at the time.

3 In 1924 the first IOSD was formed for athletes with a hearing impairment. Comité International des Sports Sourds (CISS) was a founding member of the IPC but left in 1995. Because it is currently not a member of IPC and no hearing

impaired athletes (other than those with multiple impairments who are part of the other organisations) have competed in the Paralympic Games As such this organisation is not considered of great importance in the discussion that follows.

References

Ackerman, P. L. (2014). Nonsense, common sense, and science of expert performance: Talent and individual differences. *Intelligence, 45*, 6–17.

Anderson, J. (2003). 'Turned into taxpayers': Paraplegia, rehabilitation and sport at stoke Mandeville, 1944-56. *Journal of Contemporary History, 38*(3), 461–475.

Andrews, D. L., & Silk, M. (2018). Sport and neoliberalism: An affective-ideological articulation. *Journal of Popular Culture, 51*(2), 511–533.

Baker, J., Cobley, S., Schorer, J., & Wattie, N. (2017). *The Routledge handbook of talent identification and athlete development*. London: Routledge.

Baker, J., Wattie, N., & Schorer, J. (2018). A proposed conceptualization of talent in sport: The first step in a long and winding road. *Psychology of Sport and Exercise, 43*, 27–33.

Baker, J., Wilson, S., Johnston, K., Dehghansai, N., Koenigsberg, A., de Vegt, S., et al. (2020). Talent research in sport 1990–2018: A scoping review. *Frontiers in Psychology, 11*, 607710.

Baker, J., & Young, B. W. (2020). "Talent development in sport: Moving beyond nature and nurture." In Baker, J., Cobley, S., & Schorer, J. (Eds.), *Talent identification and development in sport* (pp. 19–33). London: Routledge.

Brohm, J.-M. (1989). *Sport, A prison of measured time*. London: Pluto Press.

Colvin, G. (2010). *Talent is overrated: What really separates world-class performers from everybody else*. Penguin.

Coyle, D. (2009). *The talent code: Greatness is not born it's grown*. Bantam Books: New York

Dehghansai, N. (2021). *A comprehensive analysis of the factors affecting the development of expertise in athletes with impairments* (Publication No. 38451) [Doctoral dissertation, York University]. York Space Institutional Repository.

Dehghansai, N., & Baker, J. (2020). Searching for Paralympians: Characteristics of participants attending 'search' events. *Adapted Physical Activity Quarterly, 37*(1), 129–138.

Dehghansai, N., Pinder R. A., & Baker, J. (2021). "Looking for a golden needle in the haystack": Perspectives on talent identification and development in Paralympic sport. *Frontiers in Sports and Active Living, 3*(635977). Online publication. doi: 10.3389/fspor.2021.635977

Faris, R. E. L. (1936). Sociological factors in the development of talent and genius. *The Journal of Educational Sociology, 9*(9), 538–544.

Gladwell, M. (2008). *Outliers: The story of success*. Little, Brown.

Gruneau, R. (1999). *Class, sports and social development* (2nd ed.). Urbana, IL: Human Kinetics Press.

Guttmann, L. (1976). *Textbook of sport for the disabled*. Aylesbury. UK: HM + M Publishers.

Howe, P. D. (2008a). The tail is wagging the dog: Classification and the Paralympic movement. *Ethnography, 9*(4), 499–518.

Howe, P. D. (2008b). *The cultural politics of the Paralympic movement: Through the anthropological lens.* London: Routledge.

Howe, P. D. (2018). Athlete, anthropologist and advocate: Moving toward a life-world where difference is celebrated. *Sport and Society: Culture, Commerce, Media, Politics, 21*(4), 678–688.

Howe, P. D., & Jones, C. (2006). Classification of disabled athletes: (Dis)empowering the Paralympic practice community. *Sociology of Sport Journal, 23*(1). 29–46.

Howe, P. D., & Silva, C. F. (2018). The fiddle of using the Paralympic Games as a vehicle for expanding [dis]ability sport participation. *Sport and Society: Culture, Commerce, Media, Politics, 21*(1), 125–136.

Hughson, J. (2009). The middle class, colonialism and the making of sport. *Sport in Society, 12*(1), 69–84.

Johnston, K., Wattie, N., Schorer, J., & Baker, J. (2018). Talent identification in sport: A systematic review. *Sports Medicine, 48*(1), 97–109.

Littler, J. (2018). *Against Meritocracy: Culture, power and the myth of mobility.* London; Routledge.

Massey, W., & Whitley, M. A. (2021). The talent paradox: Disenchantment, disengagement, and damage through sport. *Sociology of Sport Journal, 38*(2), 167–177.

Morgan, W. J., (1994). *Leftist theories of sport: A critique and reconstruction.* Chicago: University of Illinois Press.

Radtke, S., & Doll-Tepper, G. (2014). *A cross-cultural comparison of talent identification and development in Paralympic sports.* Cologne: Sportverlag.

Rimmer, J., & Marques, A. C. (2012). Physical activity for people with disabilities. *The Lancet (British Edition), 380*(9838), 193–195.

Seymour, W. (1998). *Remaking the body: Rehabilitation and change.* London: Routledge.

Sheard, K., & Dunning, E. (1979). Barbarians, gentlemen and players. *A sociological study of the development of rugby football.* London: Routledge.

Silva, C. F. (2013). *The impact of sitting volleyball participation on the lives of players with impairments* (Doctoral dissertation, Loughborough University).

Silva, C. F., & Howe, P. D. (2018). The social empowerment of difference: The potential influence of Parasport. *Physical Medicine and Rehabilitation Clinics of North America, 29*(2), 397–408.

Silva, C. F., & Howe, P. D. (2019). 'Sliding to reverse ableism: An ethnographic of (Dis)ability in sitting volleyball. *Societies, 9*(41), 1–14.

INDEX

Note: Italicized and bold page numbers refer to figures and tables. Page numbers followed by "n" refer to notes.

For Product Safety Concerns and Information please contact our EU
representative GPSR@taylorandfrancis.com Taylor & Francis Verlag GmbH,
Kaufingerstraße 24, 80331 München, Germany

Printed and bound by CPI Group (UK) Ltd, Croydon, CR0 4YY

08/06/2025

01897002-0006